Maryann Papanier Wells, PhD, RN, FAAN

Surgical Instruments

A Pocket Guide

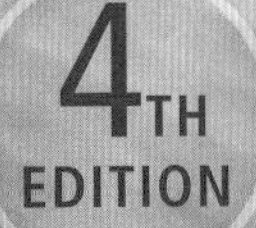

ELSEVIER
SAUNDERS

3251 Riverport Lane
St. Louis, Missouri 63043

SURGICAL INSTRUMENTS: A POCKET GUIDE

ISBN: 978-1-4377-2249-9

Notice

Neither the Publisher nor the Author assumes any re sponsibility for any loss or injury and/or damage to persons or property arising out of or related to any use of the material contained in this book. It is the responsibility of the treating practitioner, relying on independent expertise and knowledge of the patient, to determine the best treatment and method of application for the patient.

The Publisher

Library of Congress Cataloging-in-Publication Data

Wells, Maryann M. Papanier.
Surgical instruments : a pocket guide / Maryann Papanier Wells. — 4th ed.
p. ; cm.
Includes bibliographical references and index.
ISBN 978-1-4377-2249-9 (alk. paper)
1. Surgical instruments and apparatus—Handbooks, manuals, etc. I. Title.
[DNLM: 1. Surgical Instruments—Atlases. 2. Surgical Instruments—Handbooks. WO 517]
RD71.W45 2010
617'.9178—dc22

2010031278

Executive Editor: Teri Hines Burnham
Senior Developmental Editor: Laura M. Selkirk
Publishing Services Manager: Debbie Vogel
Project Manager: Beula Christopher
Cover Designer: Amy Buxton

Printed in India

Last digit is the print number: 9 8 7 6

To Allie, for always showing up and leaving your positive mark on life!

To my siblings, Karen, George and Gail, for recounting our childhood memories with the most hilarious stories!

Preface

Although patients are the focal point of operative and invasive procedures, the instruments guided by the surgeon's hand serve as the critical aspect necessary to orchestrate the ideal surgical outcome. This pocket guide was devised to support a vast array of personnel to identify the correct names of very basic instruments. It will be helpful to perioperative nurses, operating room technicians, physician assistants, medical students, instrument processing staff, central supply staff, instrument sales personnel, health care students, and educators.

This edition debuts in color, and provides a picture of each instrument in both full size and a detailed close up. The book is divided into eleven chapters, with a generic definition at the start of each section. A new chapter on Surgical Power Tools has been added. The use, varieties, and alternative names for each instrument are provided, along with space for your handwritten notes.

It takes many people to prepare a book and this was no exception. Special thanks to all of my colleagues at the Hospital of the University of Pennsylvania, from Dr. James Mullen down to the Instrument Processing staff and everyone in between who provided me with endless hours of support. *Danke* to Margaret O'Brien and Marie Zubko, who procured instruments, arranged pick ups, exchanged numerous emails and phone calls, and baby-sat photo shoots. *Tusen takk* to Michael Murphy and Frances Woodlin for their expertise regarding surgical power tools. *Mahalo* to my friends Mark Phippen, Anna Mosback, and Gerald Minardi at Covidien for supplying the endoscopic and internal stapler instrumentation. *Efcharisto poli* to the most extraordinary people, Tamara Myers and Jennifer Shropshire at Elsevier, for all of their time, camaraderie, enthusiasm, and guidance. Obrigada to Laura Selkirk and Beula Christopher for their awesome attention to detail and superb finishing touches to this book. A very appreciative *grazie mille* to Frank Pronesti and Gary Deamer for their precision and perfection in being the best photographers ever and for providing the entertainment during our numerous phone conversations.

The quote "simplicity is elegance" certainly sums up that the simpler it is, the better it is. This little pocket book continues to be a crowd pleaser, and the reception it encounters is remarkable. *Muchas gracias* to my friends and colleagues for the interest you show for this very simple book. It continues to be an honor and a privilege to be able to serve my profession. Please read, grow, and enjoy this fourth edition of *Surgical Instruments: A Pocket Guide.*

Maryann Papanier Wells, PhD, RN, FAAN

Contents

Introduction

This pocket guide examines some of the basic instruments used for operative and invasive procedures. It is divided into 11 chapters.

Chapter 1, Sharps/Dissectors/Cutting, reviews chisels, curettes, bone cutters, elevators, knives, mallets, osteotomes, rasps, rongeurs, saws, scissors, snares, and trephines. Chapter 2, Forceps/Grasping, reviews smooth, toothed, bayonet, and bipolar forceps. Chapter 3, Clamps/Holding, reviews a variety of clamps. Chapter 4, Retractors, reviews self-retaining and handheld retractors used for superficial to deep wound surgical specialties. Chapter 5, Suture Devices/Needle Holders, reviews all types of needle holders, ranging from very fine to very heavy tips, and ligating clip appliers. Chapter 6, Suction Tips, reviews suction tips of various dimensions and widths from micro to macro. Chapter 7, Dilators/Probes, reviews a variety of dilators. Chapter 8, Minimally Invasive Surgical Instruments, reviews various types of endoscopic instruments used for both laparoscopic and robotic surgical specialties. Chapter 9, Internal Staplers, reviews the various kinds of anastomotic staple devices used for open surgical procedures. Chapter 10, Surgical Power Tools, reviews various types of both battery operated and nitrogen operated power tools. Chapter 11, Routine Instrument Sets, offers the contents necessary to compile minor, major, endoscopic, laparoscopic, or robotic instruments sets. Refer to the glossary for basic definitions.

Photo Credits

All images included in *Surgical Instruments: A Pocket Guide* were photographed by Frank Pronesti of Heirloom Studio.

Frank Pronesti
www.heirloomstudio.com
Heirloom Studio
40 S. Main St.
Yardley, PA 19067
215-321-9559

Reviewers

Angela Arrington, ST
Surgical Technician
Delaware County Community College Alumni
Media, Pennsylvania

Connie Bell, CST
National Surgical Technology Program Director
Glendale Career College
Glendale, California

Rae Fierro, RN, CNOR, RNFA
Charge Nurse, Outpatient Surgery
Jefferson Surgical Center
Philadelphia, Pennsylvania

Patricia Greco, CST
Certified Surgical Technologist
Berwyn, Pennsylvania

Rachel Hottel, MSN, RN, CNOR
Advanced Practice Nurse, PeriOperative Division
University of Iowa Hospitals and Clinics
Iowa City, Iowa

Karen E. Lipinski
CSTFA
Mercy Medical Center
Sioux City, Iowa

Leigh W. Moore, MSN, RN, CNOR, CNE
Associate Professor of Nursing, ADN Program
Southside Virginia Community College
Alberta, Virginia

Michael Murphy, MSN, RN
Clinical Educator, Perioperative Nursing
Hospital of the University of Pennsylvania
Philadelphia, Pennsylvania

Tera Pape, PhD, RN, CNOR
Associate Professor, College of Nursing – Denton Campus
Texas Woman's University
Denton, Texas

Barbara Putrycus, RN, MSN
Director
Infection Control, Quality, Regulatory Compliance/Surgical Services
Oakwood Hospital and Medical Center
Dearborn, Michigan

Vanetta Cheeks Reeder, RN, MSN, CNOR
Nurse Educator, Perioperative Services
Hospital of the University of Pennsylvania
Philadelphia, Pennsylvania

Catherine Napoli Rice, EdD, RN
Professor of Nursing
Western Connecticut State University
Danbury, Connecticut

Susan Rico, RN, BSN
Service Manager of Vascular Surgery
The Louis Stokes VA Medical Center
Cleveland, Ohio

Diane Saullo, RN, BSN, MSN, CNOR, BC
Manager, Professional Development Department
New Hanover Regional Medical Center
Wilmington, North Carolina

Nancy Venezia, RN, AAS
Registered Nurse
Chestnut Hill Hospital
Philadelphia, Pennsylvania

CHAPTER 1

Sharps/Dissectors/Cutting

Sharps are instruments used to cut, dissect, incise, separate, or excise tissue. They may have sharp or blunt edges. They are also known as mechanical cutters.

2

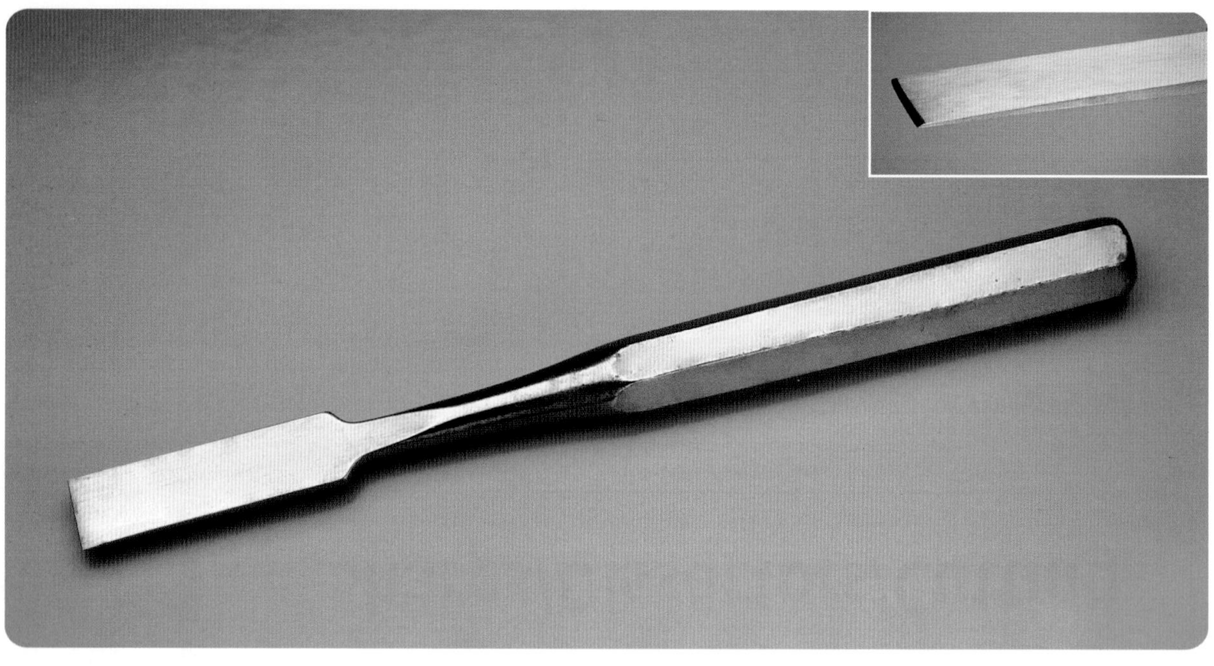

Chisel/Bone

USE • To sculpt bone; to aid in cutting a bone graft; to use with a mallet

VARIETIES • 6 ½ or 8 inches long; various widths between 4 and 25 mm

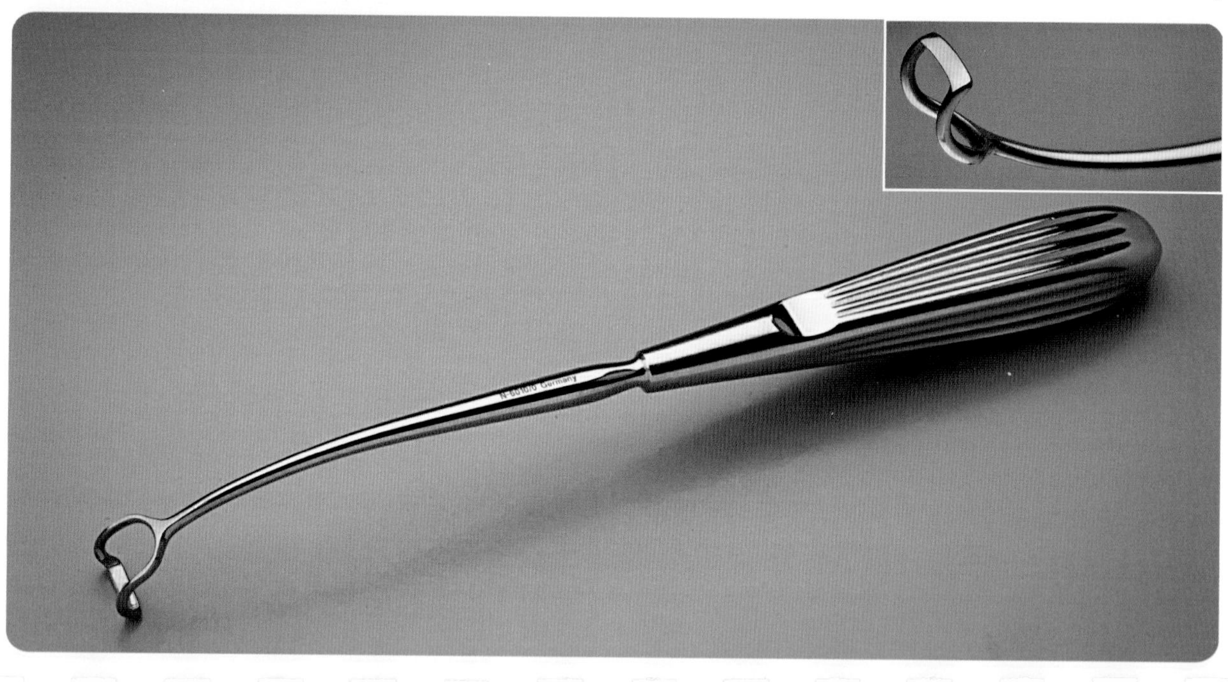
Germany

Curette/Adenoid

USE • To scrape remnants of adenoid tissue

VARIETIES • Approximately 8½ inches long with curette openings ranging from 6 to 21 mm wide and 15 to 30 mm long; some are angled

ALSO KNOWN AS • Barnhill curette, Stubbs curette, Vogel curette

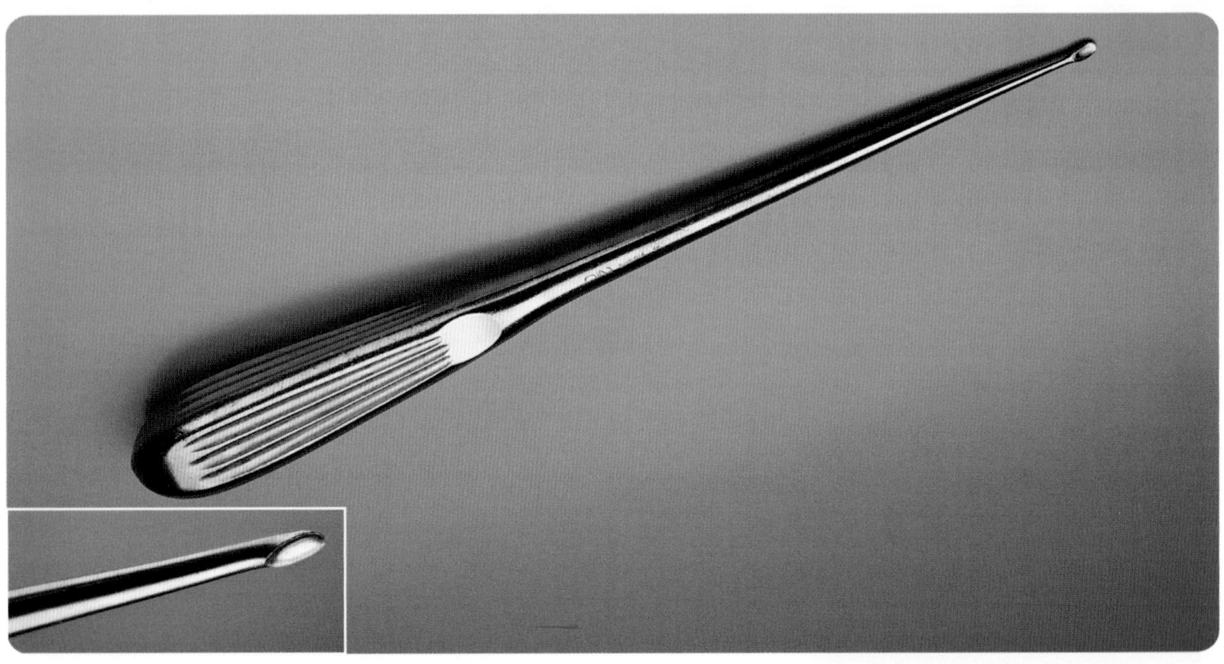

9

Curette/Bone

USE • To scrape bone; to debride tissue; to scoop tissue out of small areas; to scoop cancellous bone for grafting

VARIETIES • Angled or straight; open or cupped; various sizes

ALSO KNOWN AS • Brun curette

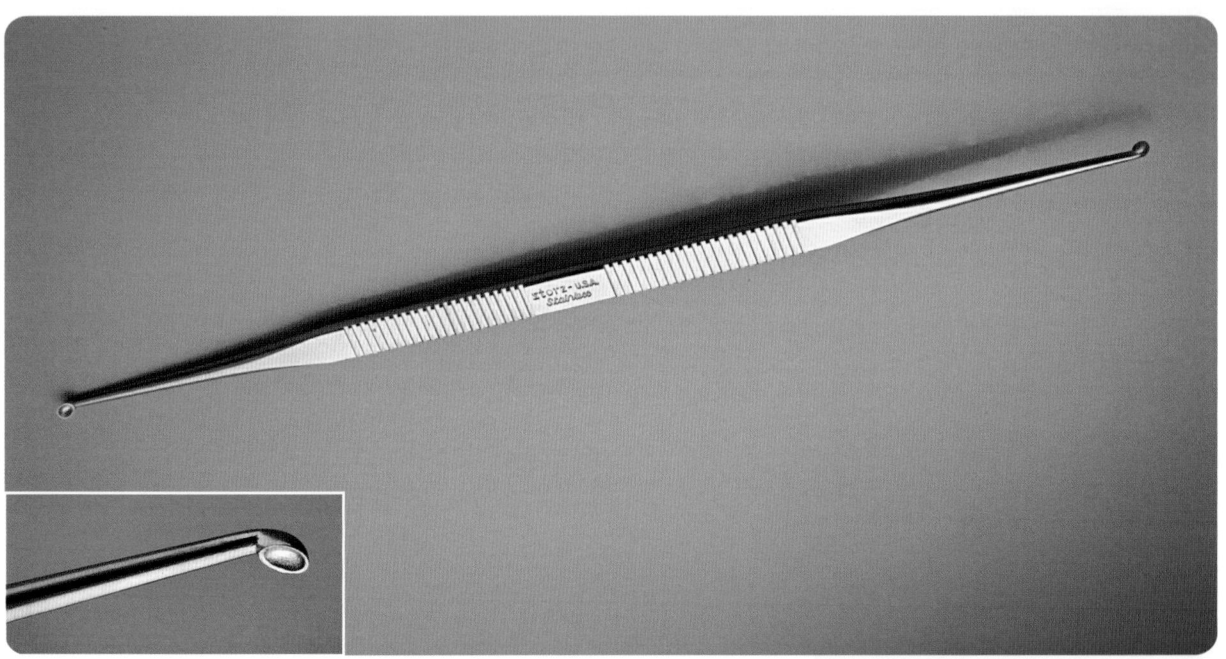

8

Curette/Dermal

USE • To scrape dermis

VARIETIES • Open, hook-shaped end, ring end, or cup shape; 3 to 6 mm wide

ALSO KNOWN AS • Fox dermal curette, Myles antrum curette, ring curette, Walsh dermal curette

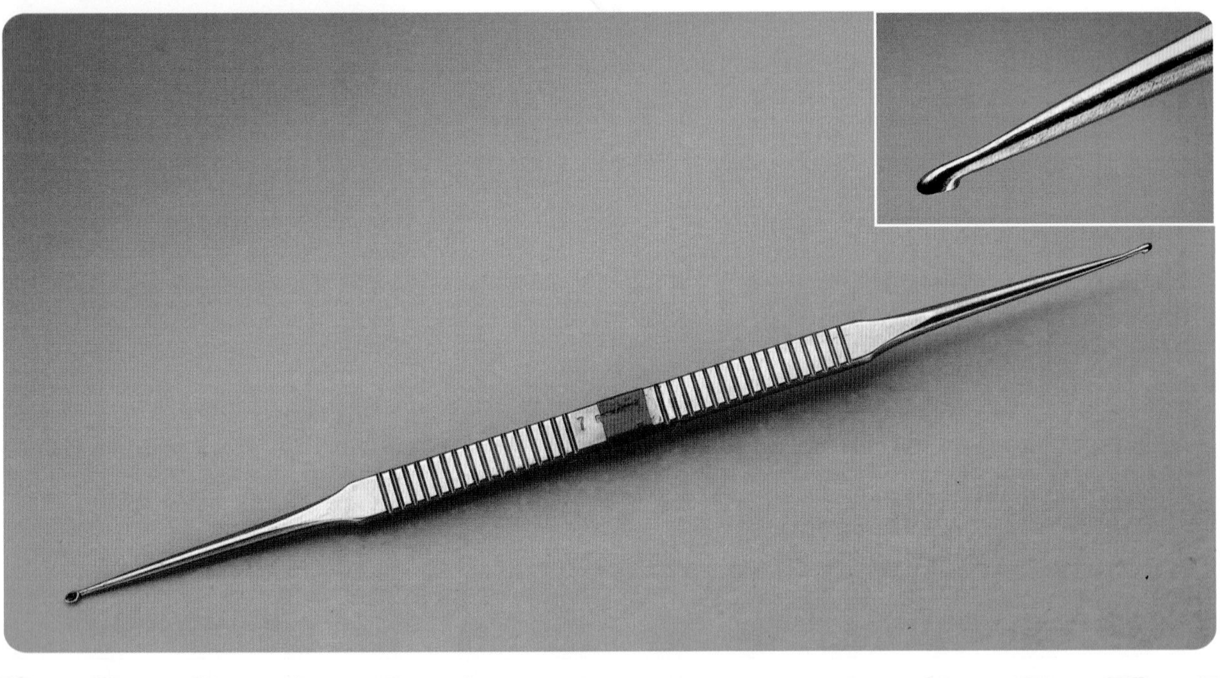

Curette/Ear

USE • To scrape inner ear (i.e., stapes); to remove debris from ear canal

VARIETIES • Single- or double-ended oval or round cups; sharp or blunt, sizes 00 to 3 mm

ALSO KNOWN AS • Billeau curette, Buck curette, ear loop, Shapleigh curette

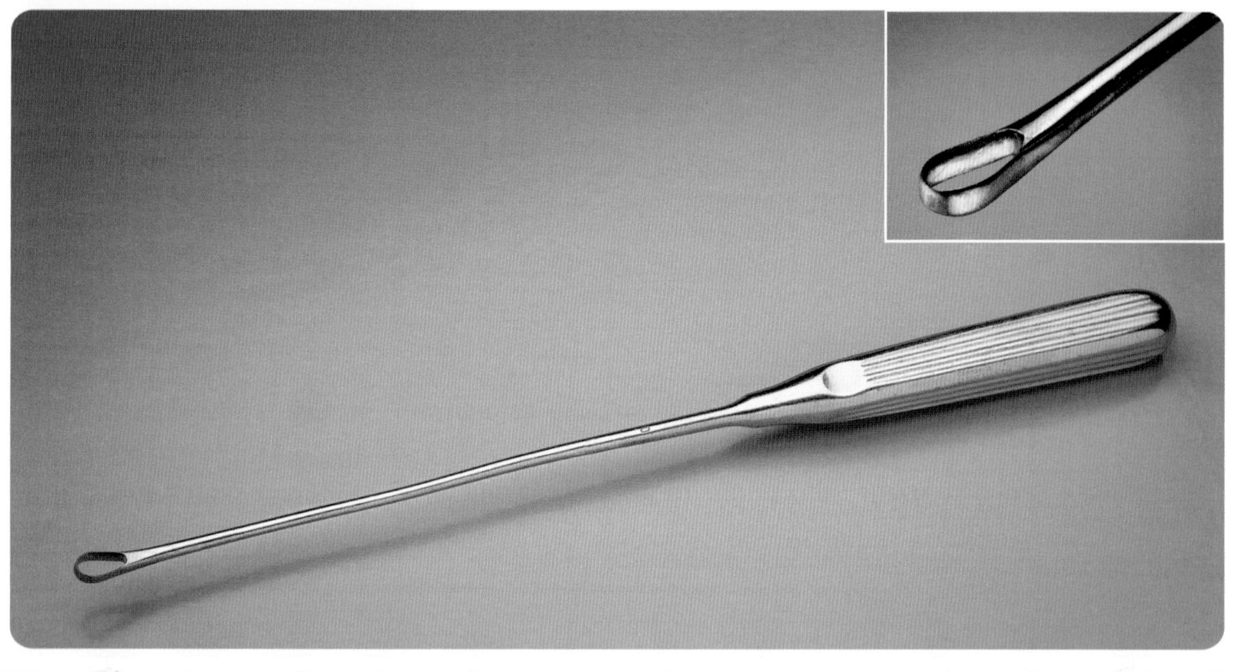

Curette/Uterine

USE • To scrape endometrial lining of uterus; to roughen up tissue in a nonhealing wound to enhance secondary closure

VARIETIES • Serrated cutting edge; open ring, 9½ inches long

ALSO KNOWN AS • Heaney uterine curette

14

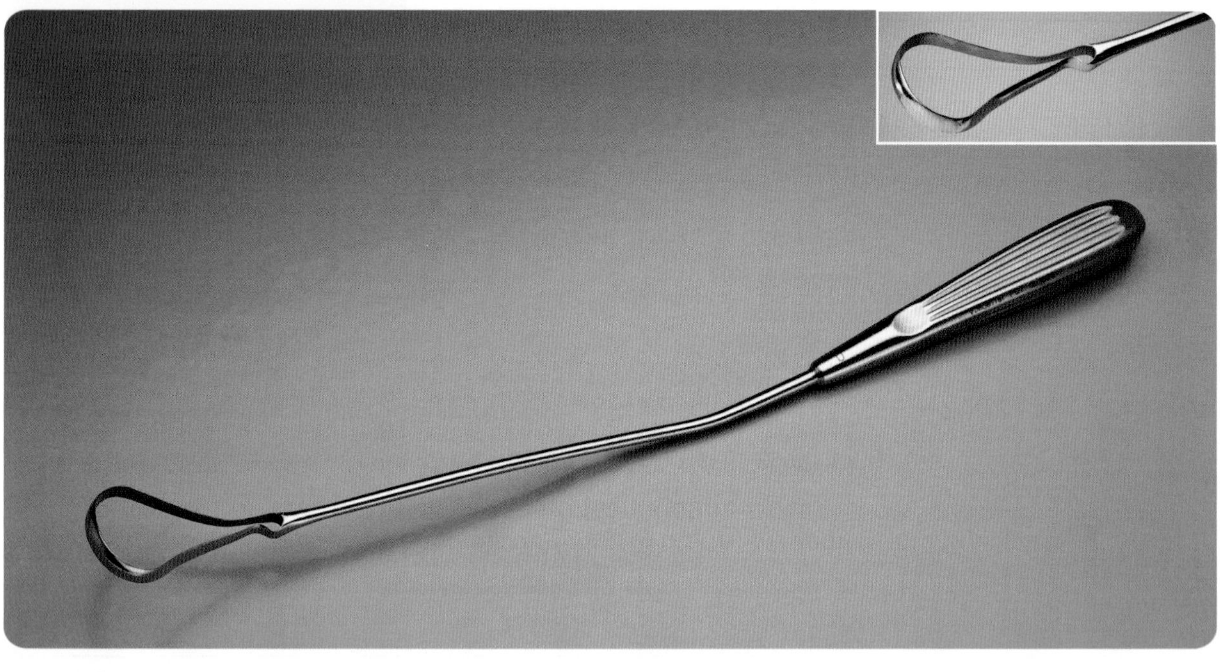

Curette/Uterine, Large

USE • To scrape uterine cavity (usually postpregnancy uterus)

VARIETIES • Large, open ring; blade 3 cm wide

ALSO KNOWN AS • Hunter curette, Hunter uterine curette

16

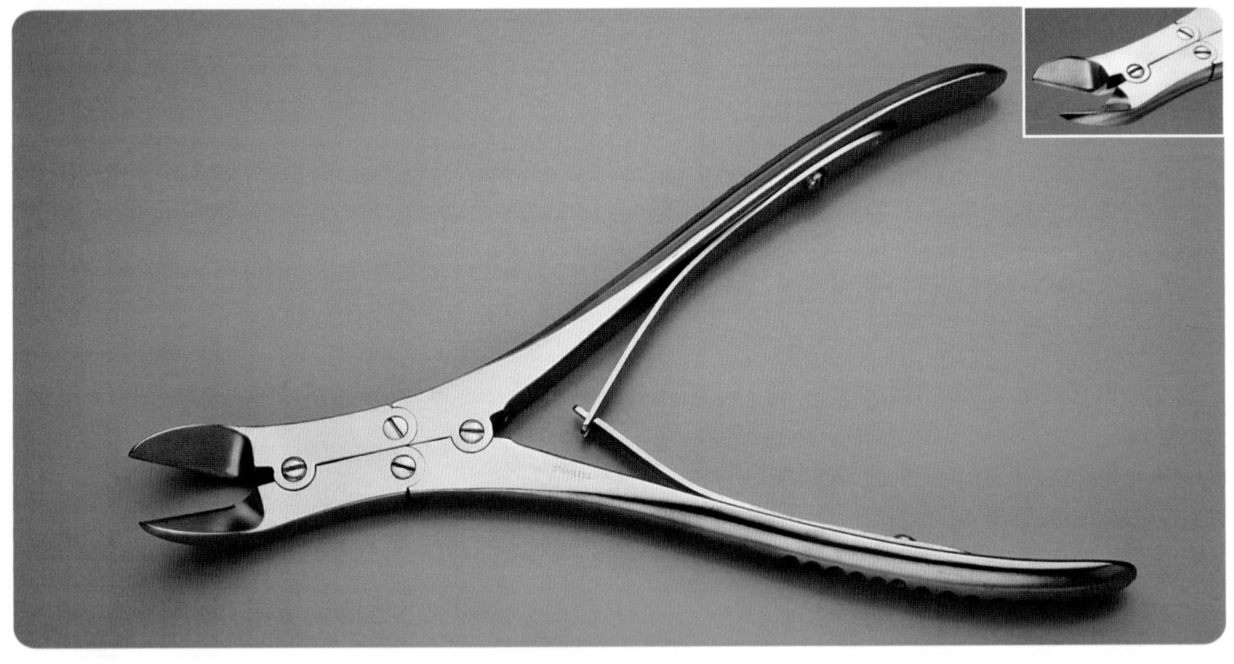

Cutter/Bone

USE • To cut bone and cartilage

VARIETIES • Straight or curved; single or double action; straight or angled jaw

ALSO KNOWN AS • Bone biter, Liston bone cutting forceps, rib shears

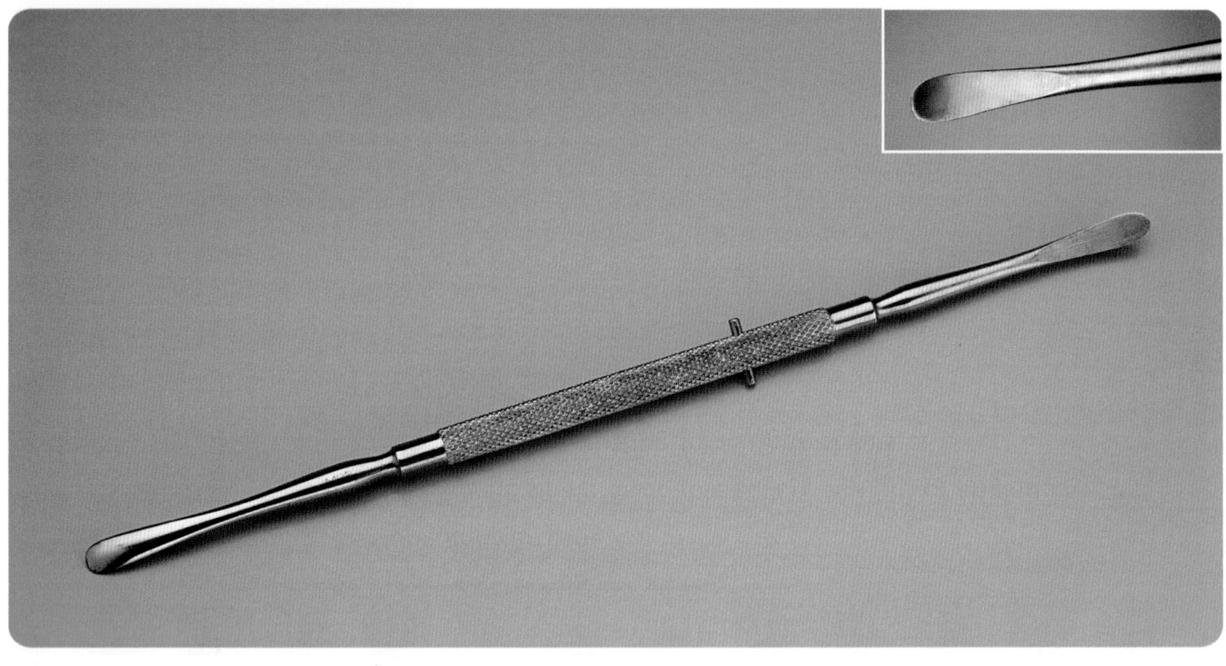

Elevator/Freer

USE • To take tissue off cartilage (e.g., nasal septum); to scrape plaque from large arteries in cardiovascular procedures; to lift periosteum from bone in orthopedic procedures; to press small balls of bone wax onto bone edges for hemostasis in neurosurgery procedures

VARIETIES • Double-ended; sharp or blunt blades, 7 inches long

ALSO KNOWN AS • Cottle elevator, Pierce elevator

20

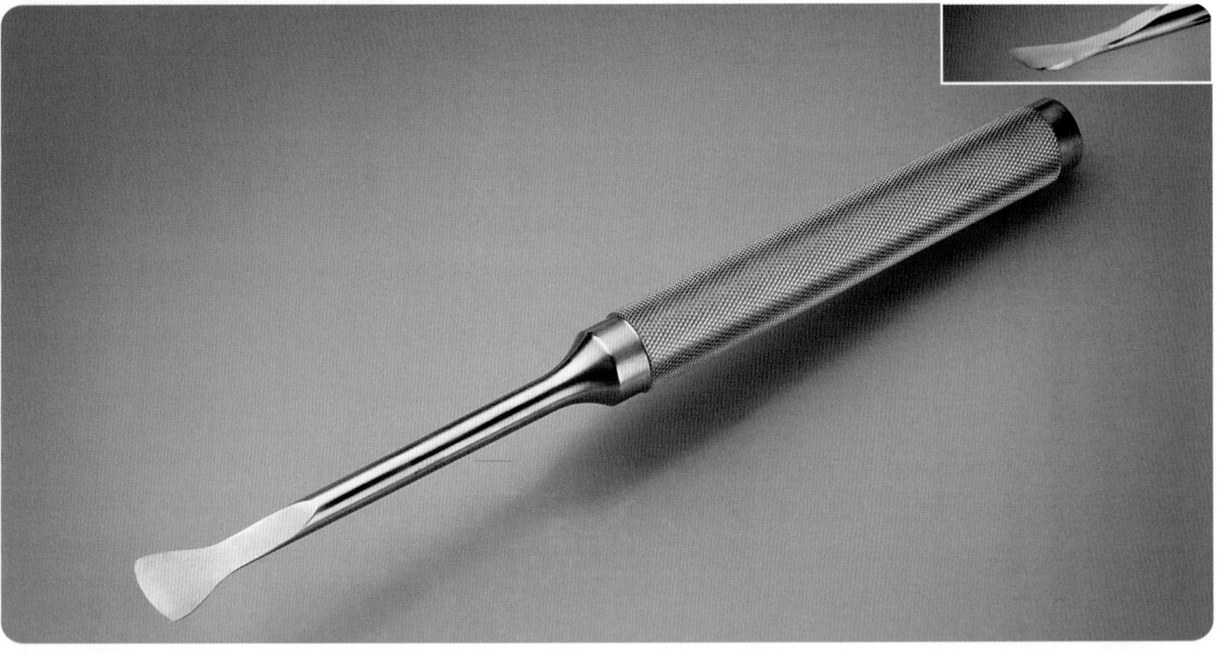

Elevator/Periosteal

USE • To scrape and remove periosteum from bone in preparation for a bone incision

VARIETIES • Single- or double-ended; sharp or blunt; curved or straight; narrow or wide

ALSO KNOWN AS • Chandler elevator, Cobb elevator, converse elevator, Farabeuf elevator, Joseph elevator, key elevator, Langenbeck elevator, Penfield elevator, Sayre elevator

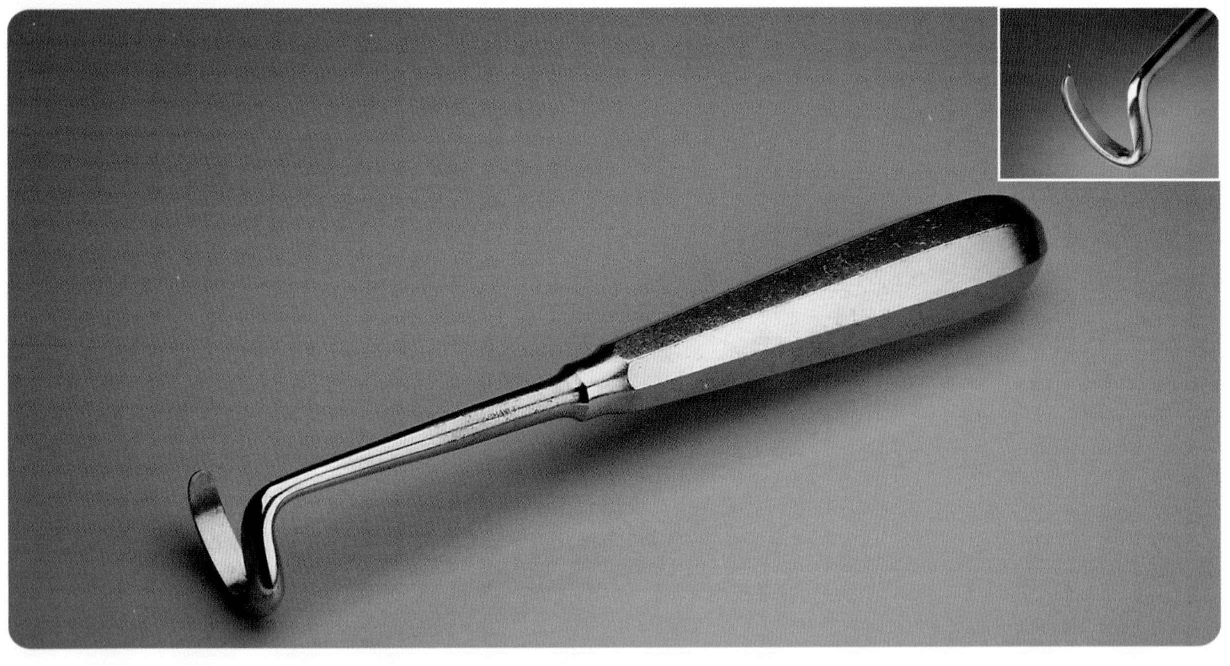

Elevator/Rib

USE • To scrape along ribs to remove tissue and cartilage

VARIETIES • Right or left blade; pediatric and adult sizes

ALSO KNOWN AS • Doyen raspatory, Doyen rib elevator, rib stripper and elevator

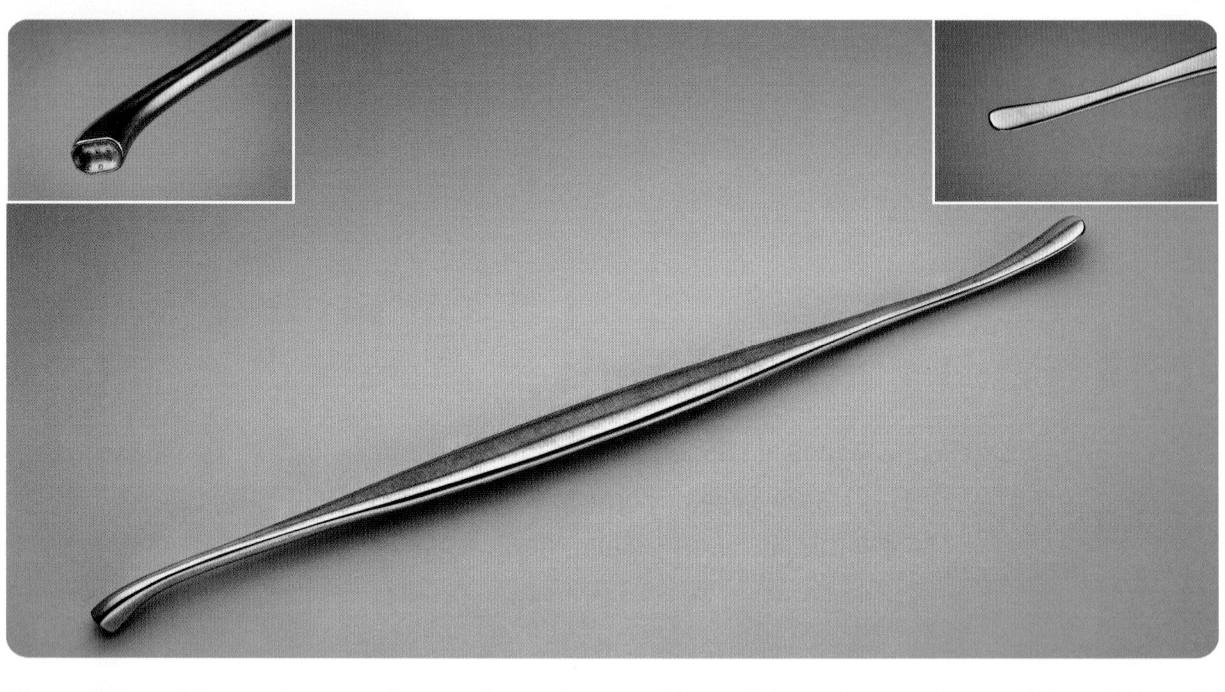

Elevator/Septum

USE • To elevate and dissect septum during intranasal procedures; to dissect nerve vessels and bone in neurosurgical procedures; to use as a bone wax tamp

VARIETIES • Single-ended with blunt blade

ALSO KNOWN AS • Cottle elevator, Freer elevator

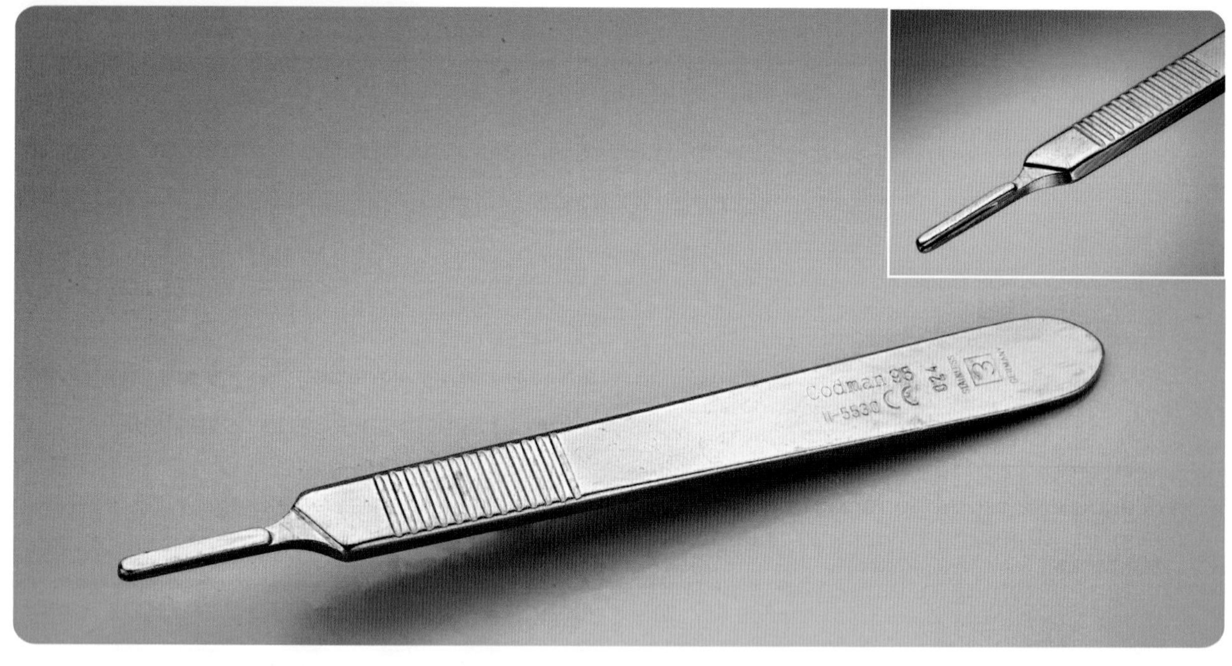

Handle/Scalpel

USE • To accommodate knife blades of many sizes (e.g., #10, #15, #11)

VARIETIES • Various lengths from short to long; usually straight but can be angled

ALSO KNOWN AS • Cutter, knife, knife handle

28

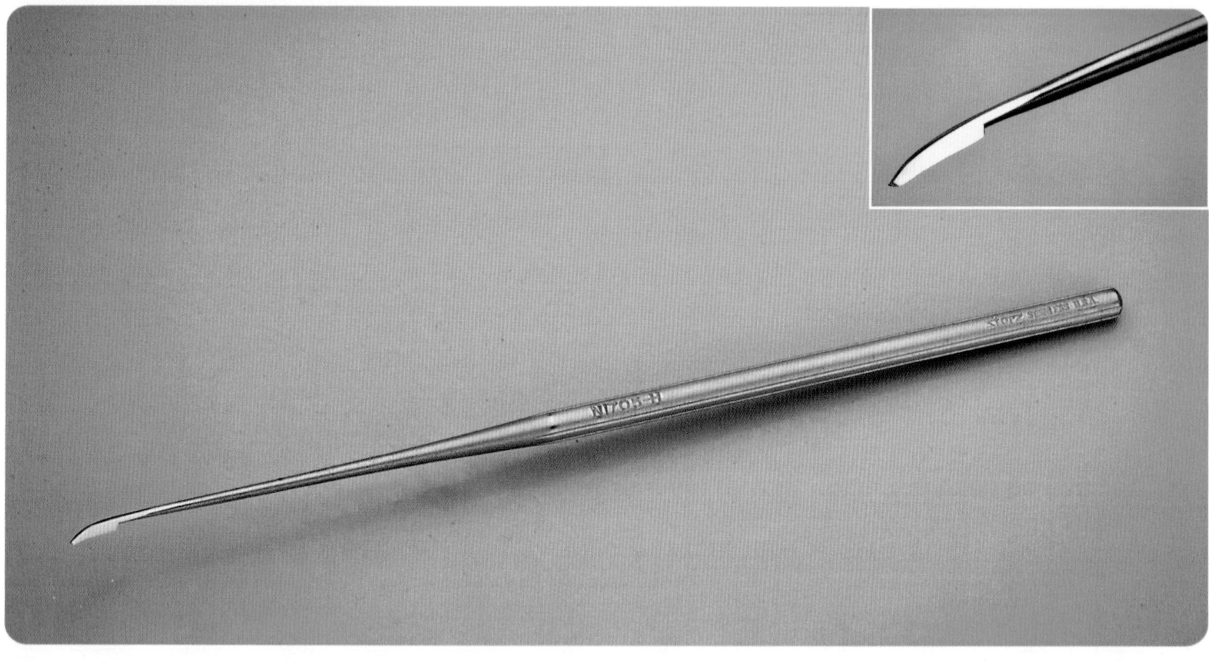

Knife/Ear

USE • To create a fine puncture in the tympanic membrane for ear drainage in myringotomy

VARIETIES • Reusable or disposable; straight blade, 6½ or 7 inches long

ALSO KNOWN AS • Myringotomy knife, Sexton ear knife

30

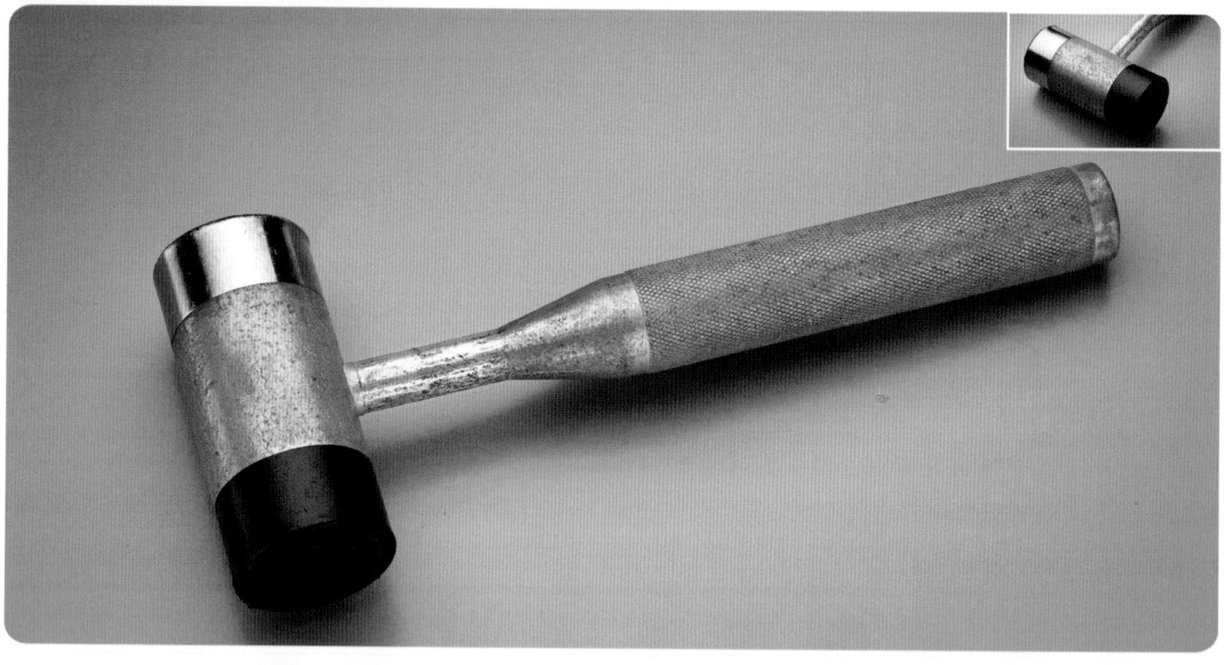

Mallet

USE • To exert force on an object (e.g., to drive a nail into a bone); to use a chisel or osteotome as a guide

VARIETIES • Several sizes, weights, and lengths

ALSO KNOWN AS • Cooper mallet, Cottle mallet, Gerzog mallet, hammer, Lucae mallet, Mead mallet, Peck mallet

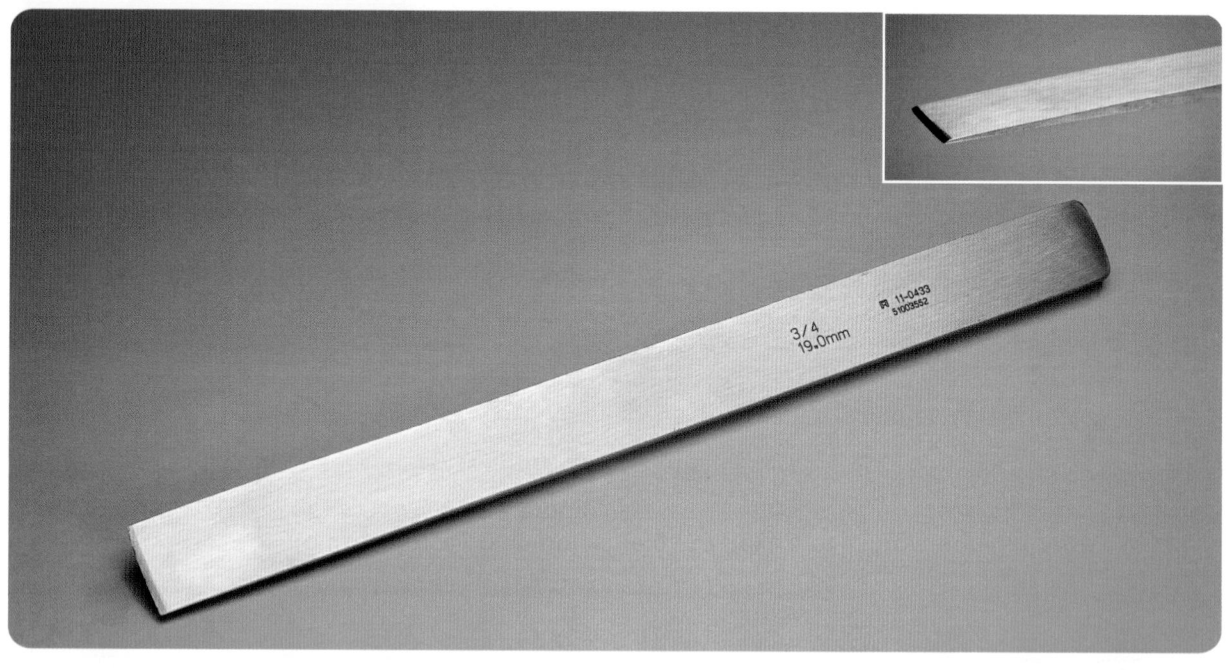
3/4
19.0mm
11-0433
51003552

Osteotome/Lambotte

USE • To score or place cuts in bone

VARIETIES • Curved or straight; 9 inches long; 6, 13, 19, 25, 32, or 38 mm wide

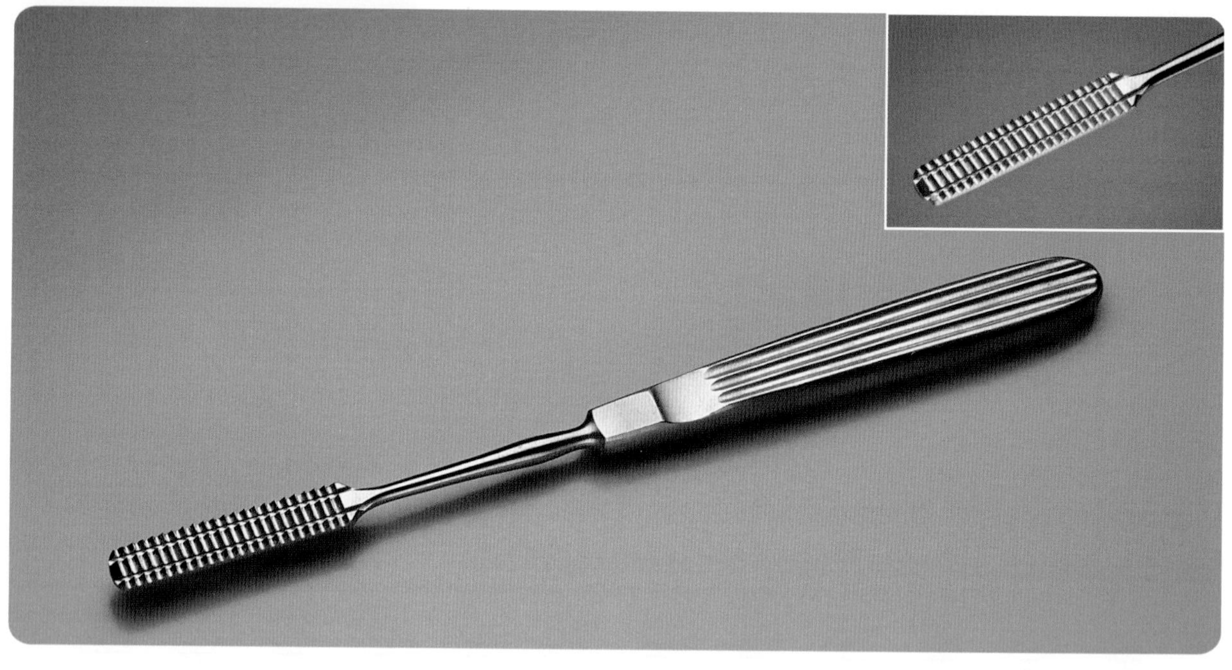

Rasp

USE • To smooth a rough bone surface or to evacuate medullary canals in preparation for prosthesis insertion

VARIETIES • Single- or double-ended; curved or tapered blades, forward and backward cutting; fine or coarse teeth

ALSO KNOWN AS • Aufricht rasp, Cottle rasp, Fomon rasp, Lewis rasp, Maltz rasp, Putti rasp, Wiener rasp

36

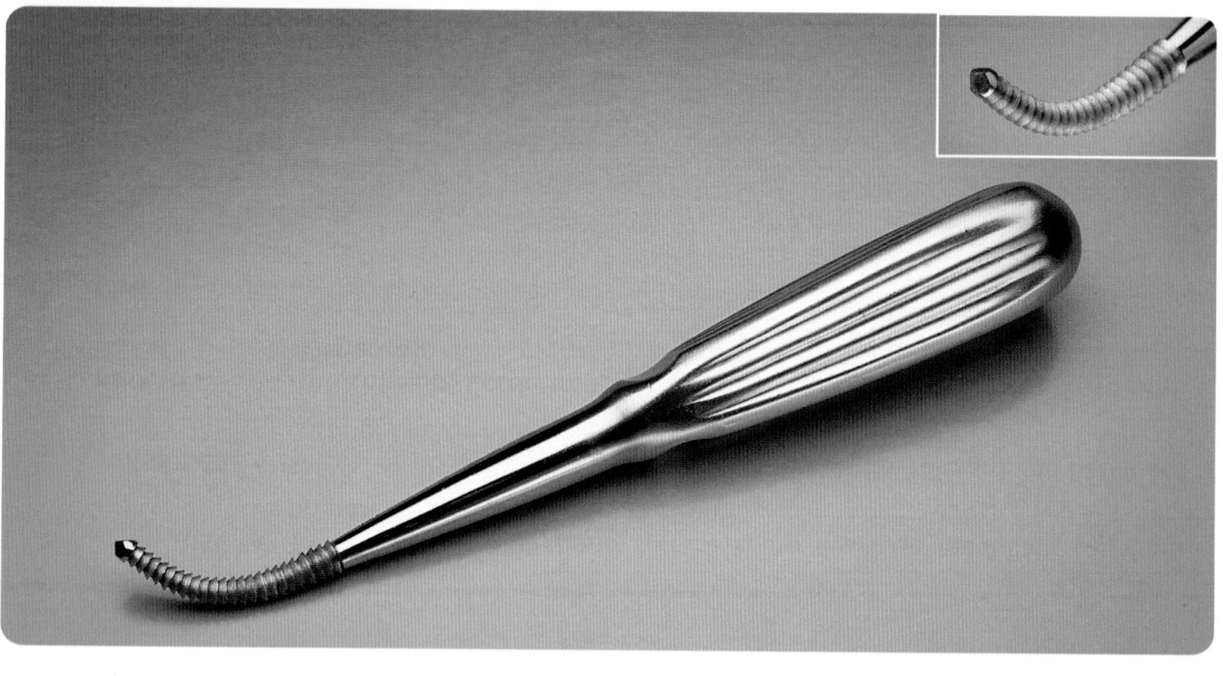

Rasp/Nasal, Wiener

USE • To mechanically smooth nasal cartilage and bone during septoplasty

VARIETIES • Small, medium, and large with trocar tips

ALSO KNOWN AS • Wiener antral rasp

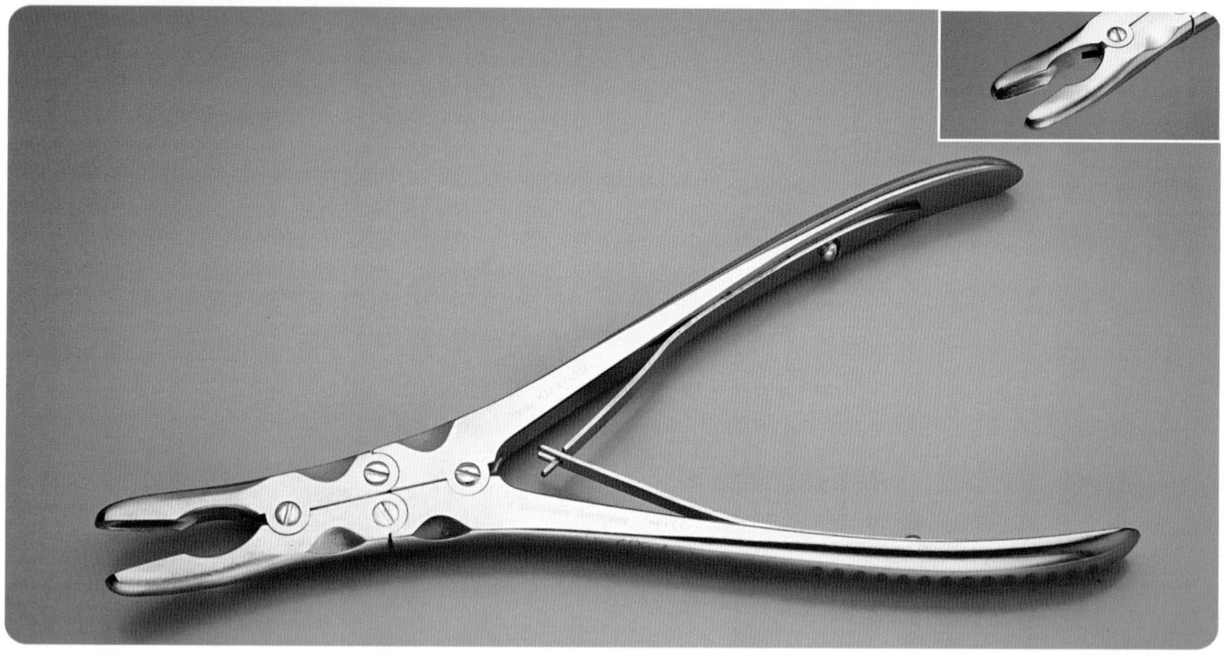

Rongeur/Double-Action

USE • To cut through small segments of bone

VARIETIES • Curved or straight jaws; 4 to 8 mm bite

ALSO KNOWN AS • Beyer rongeur, Jansen-Zaufel rongeur, Leksell rongeur, Luer-Echlin rongeur, Ruskin rongeur, Stille rongeur

40

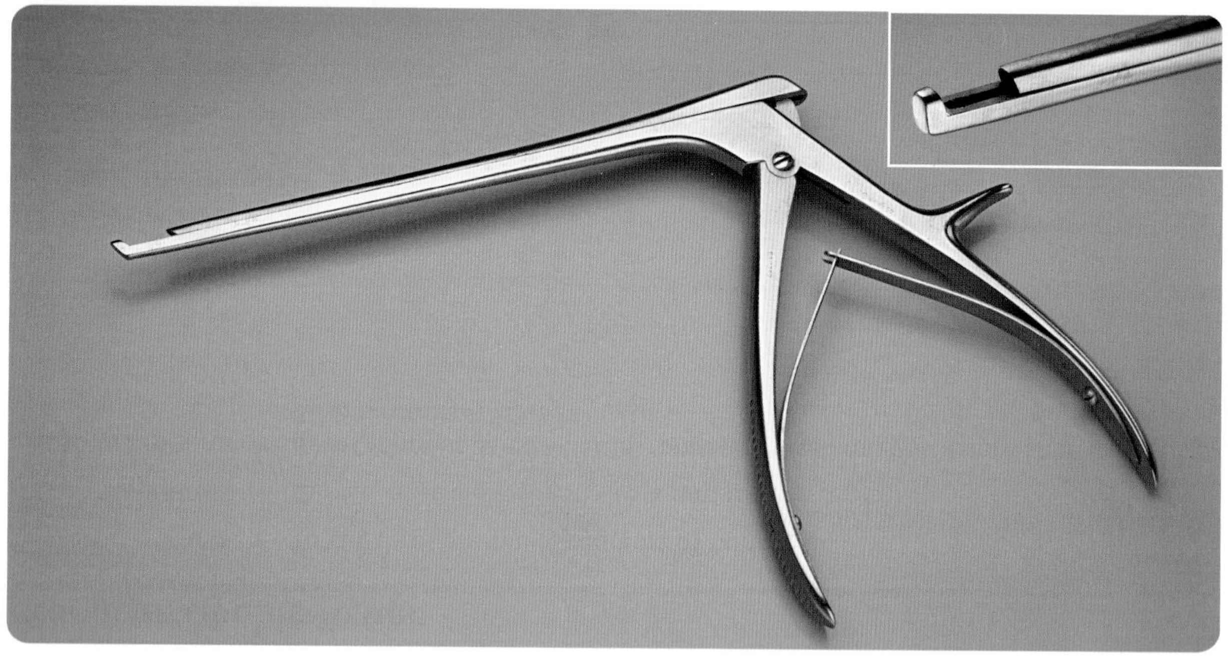

Rongeur/Kerrison

USE • To remove delicate bones during neurosurgery (e.g., laminectomy) and orthopedic procedures

VARIETIES • Up or down biting; 90 or 40 degree angled jaw; 3.5 to 6.5 mm bite

ALSO KNOWN AS • Up bite, down bite

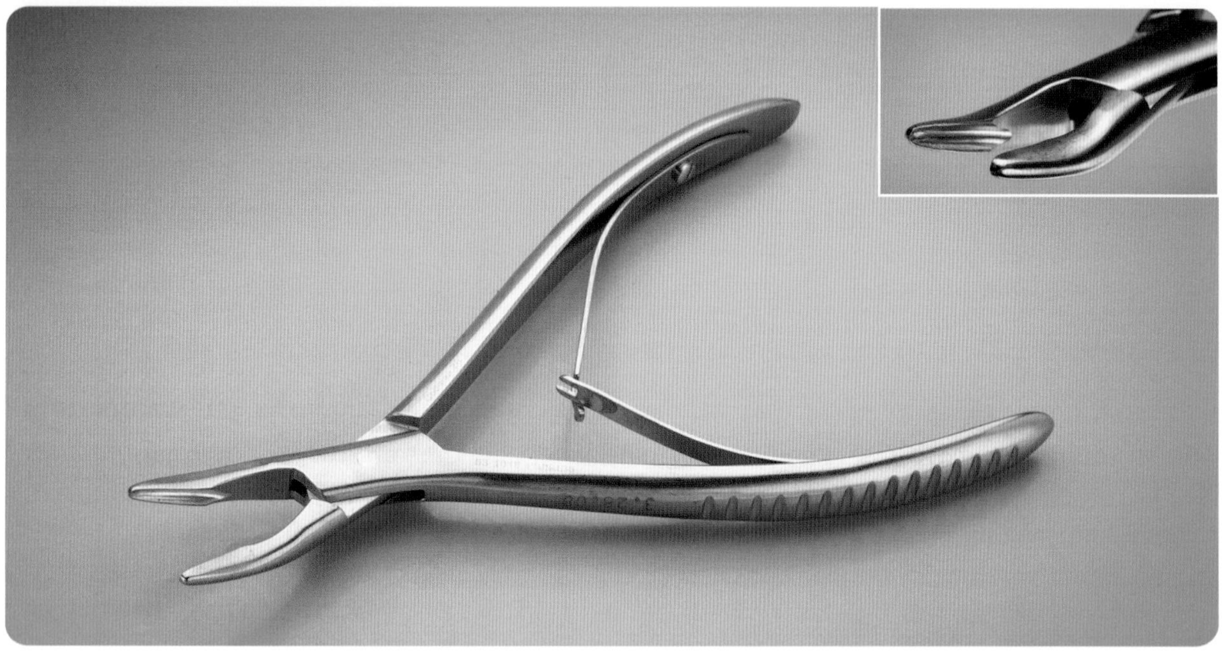

Rongeur/Lempert

USE • To remove bone; to remove soft tissue from around bone

VARIETIES • Straight; curved; delicate; 2.5 mm bite

ALSO KNOWN AS • Juers-Lempert rongeur

44

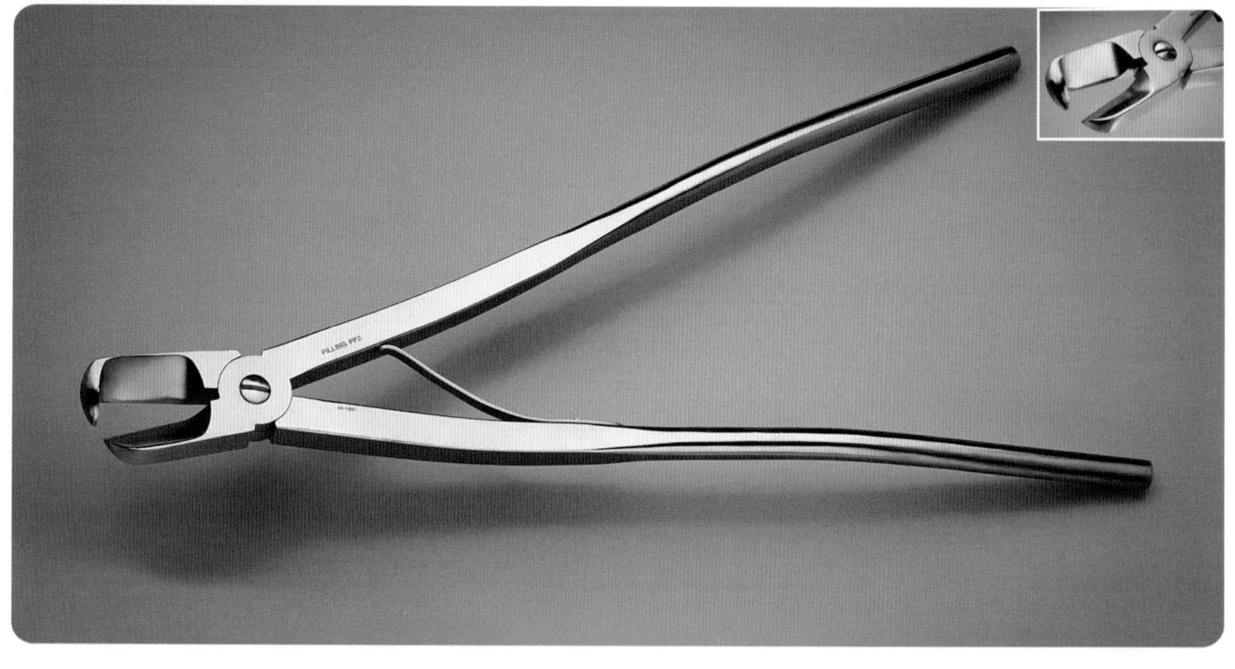

Rongeur/Rib

USE • To cut ribs

VARIETIES • Right- or left-oriented; pediatric and adult sizes

ALSO KNOWN AS • Bethune rongeur, Coryllos rongeur, rib cutter, rib shears, Sauerbruch rongeur

46

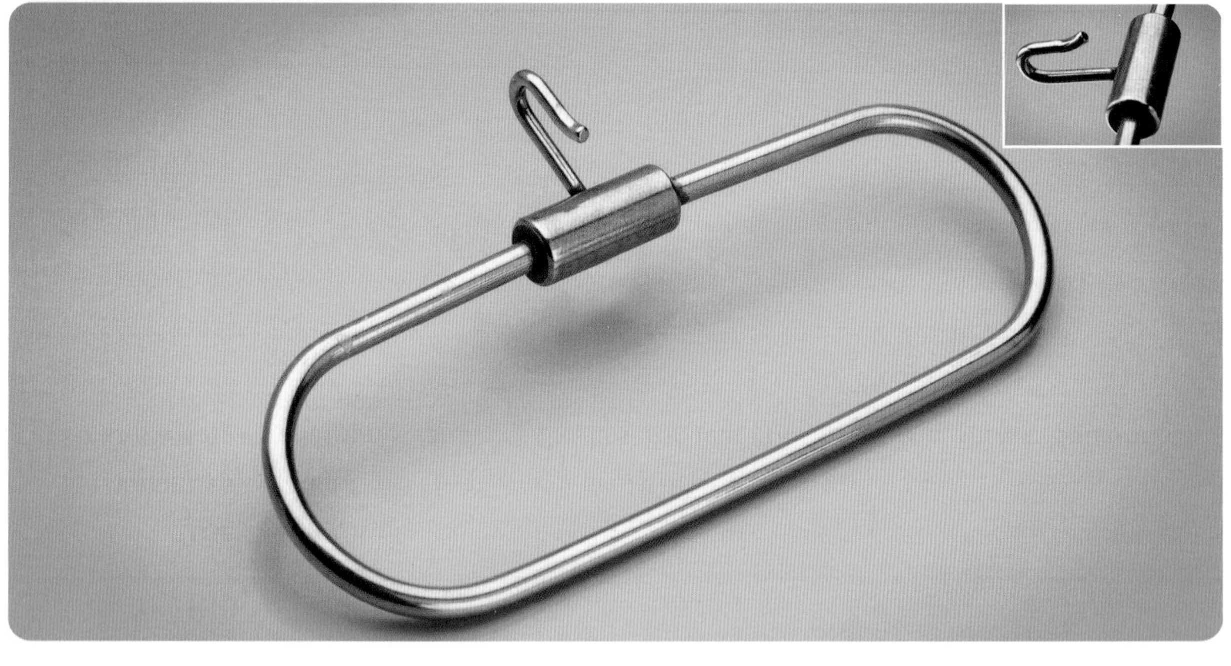

Saw/Gigli, Handle for

USE • To hold Gigli saw blade for controlled severing of bone during amputation

VARIETIES • Standard size

48

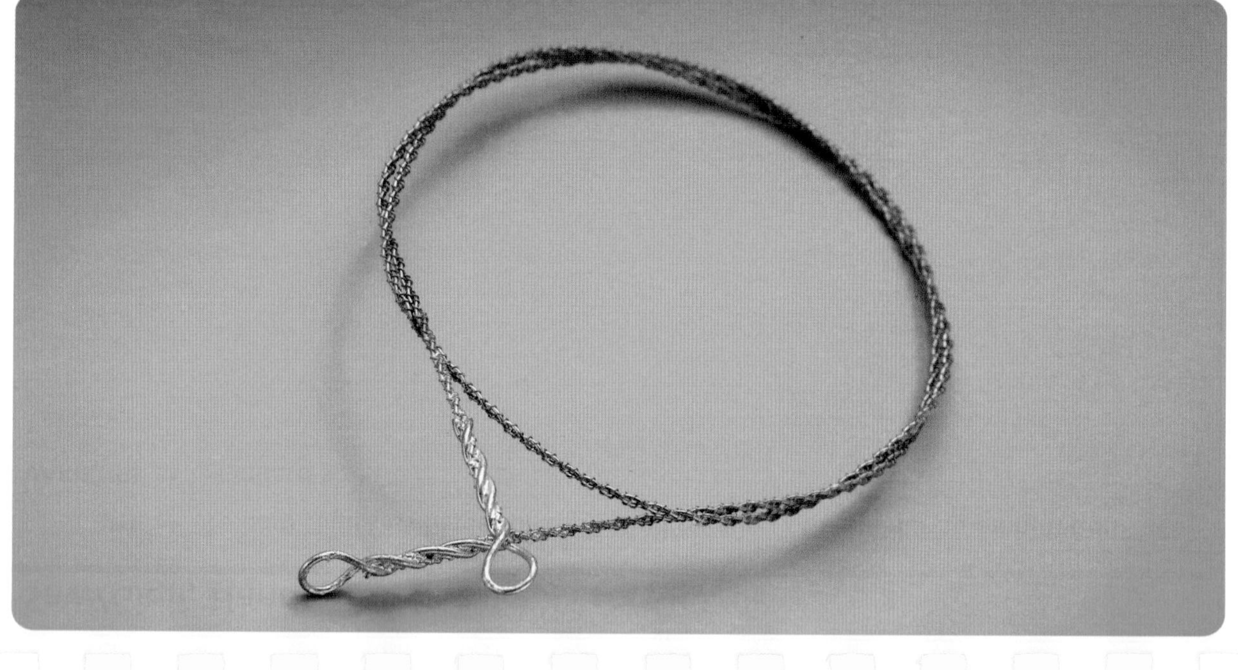

Saw/Gigli, Wire Blade for

USE • To cut small and large bone during amputation

VARIETIES • 12 or 20 inches long

ALSO KNOWN AS • Amputation wire

50

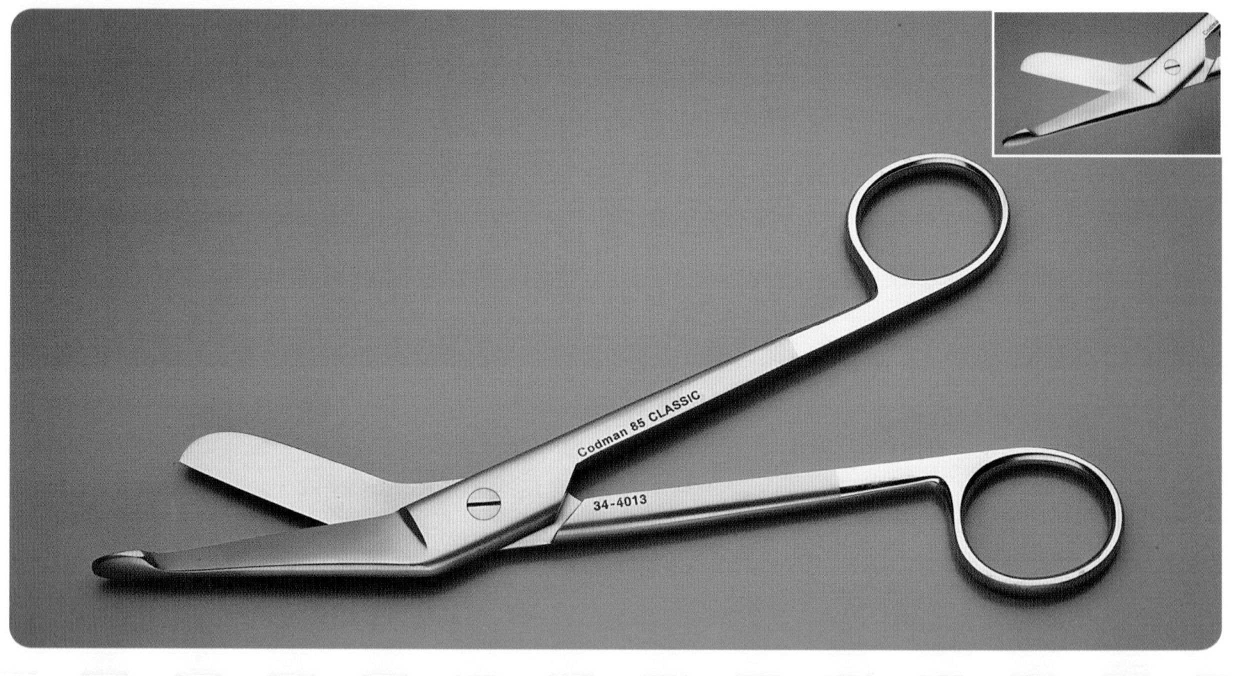

Scissors/Bandage

USE • To cut bandages and dressings; to open uterus during a C-section

VARIETIES • Angled blades with unilateral blunted tip; various lengths

ALSO KNOWN AS • Esmarch scissors, Lister scissors, tape scissors

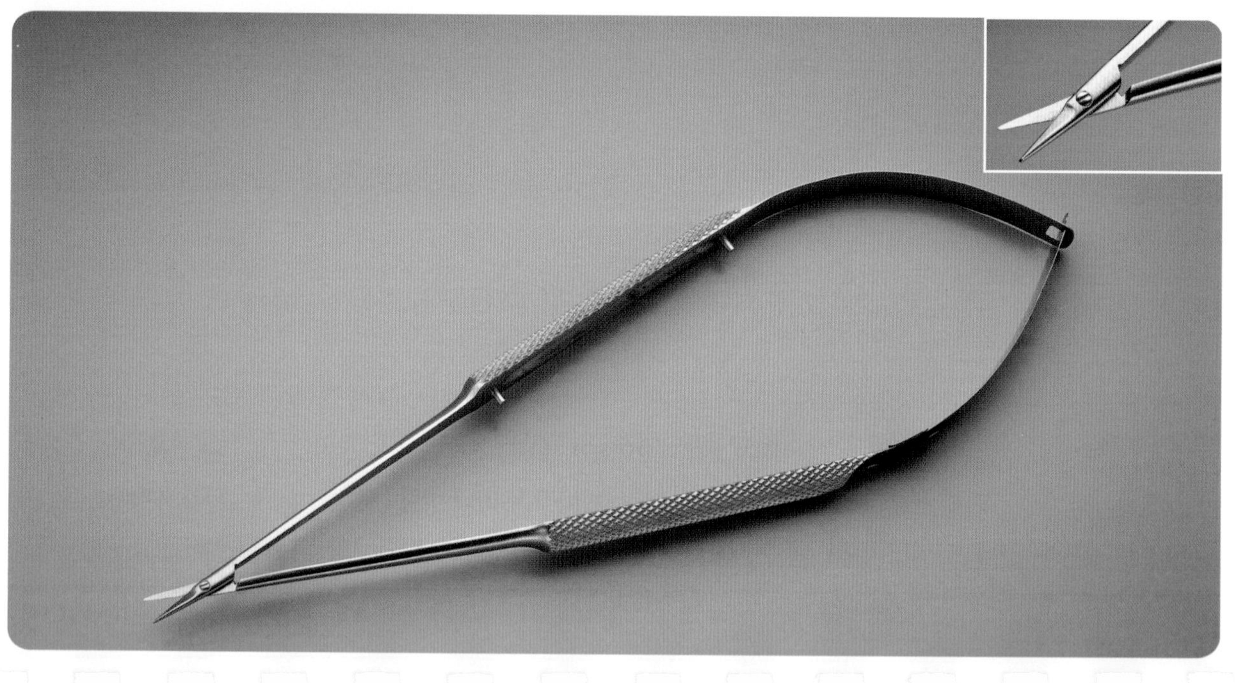

Scissors/Castroviejo

USE • To cut tissue during fine (e.g., microvascular) dissection; to extend an arterotomy or venotomy

VARIETIES • Fine, spring-operated blades; short or long; straight or curved; right or left oriented

ALSO KNOWN AS • Microscissors

54

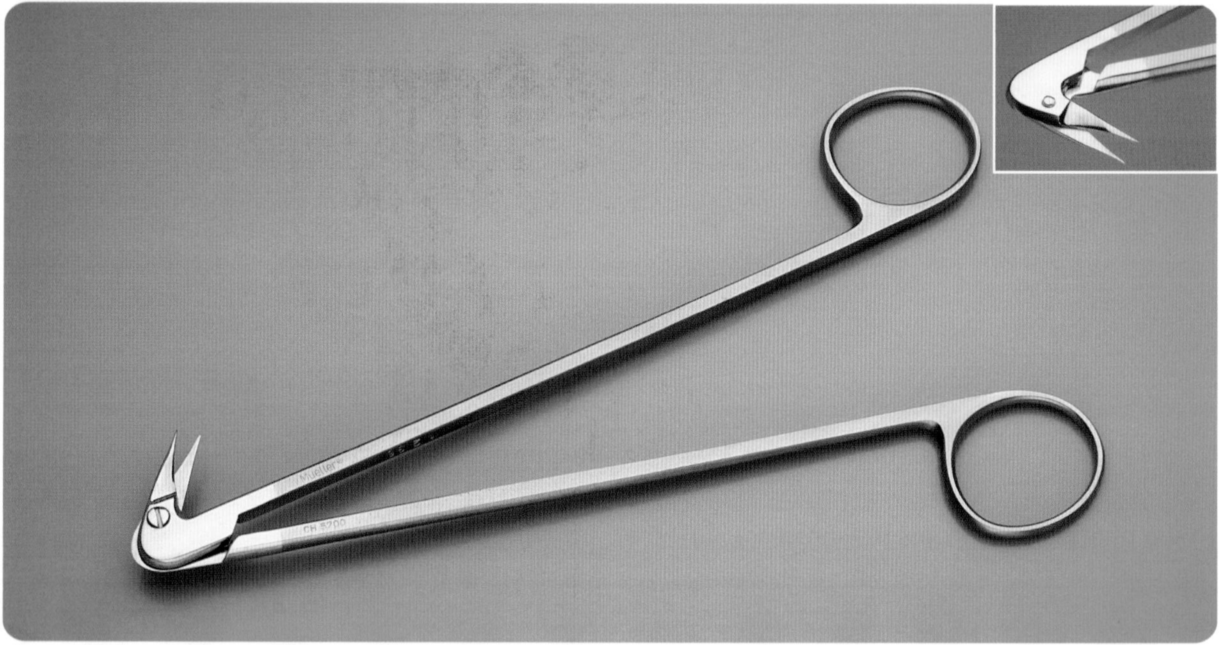

Scissors/Circumflex

USE • To cut vascular tissue during open heart procedure; to extend a coronary artery

VARIETIES • Angled blades

ALSO KNOWN AS • Beall scissors, Mills scissors

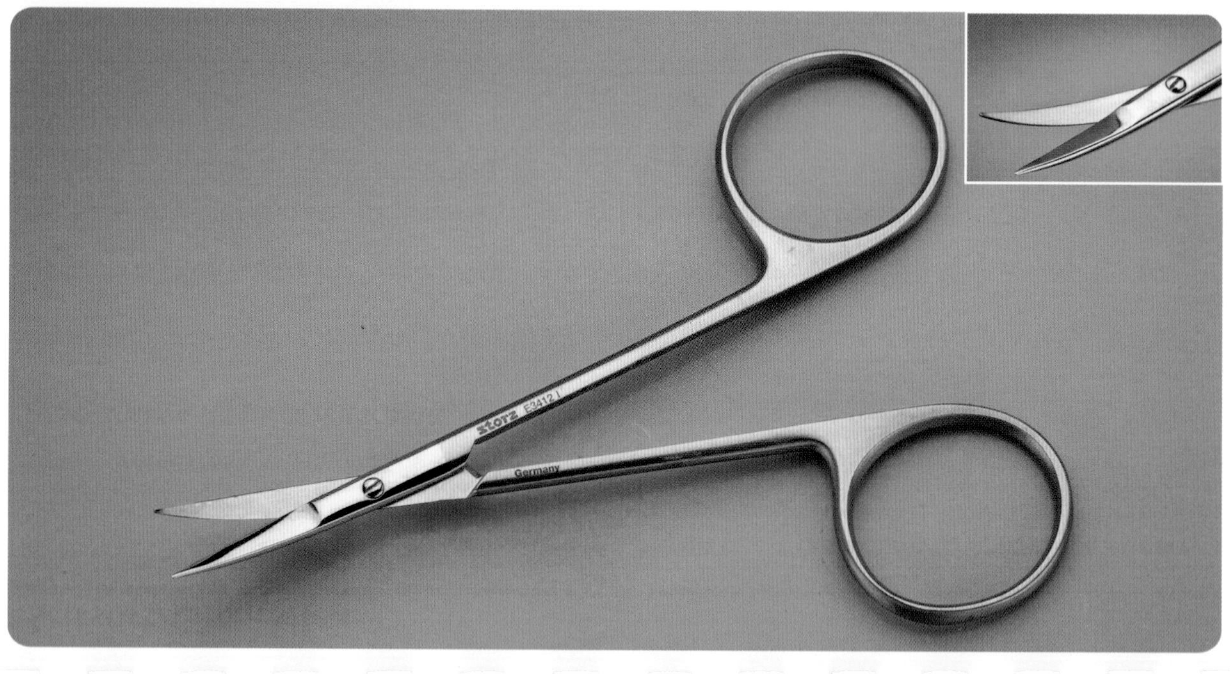
storz E3412 I
Germany

Scissors/Iris

USE • To cut delicate tissue during plastic, hand, and minor vascular surgery

VARIETIES • Small, fine sharp/sharp blades; straight or curved; 4 ½ inches long

ALSO KNOWN AS • Plastic scissors

58

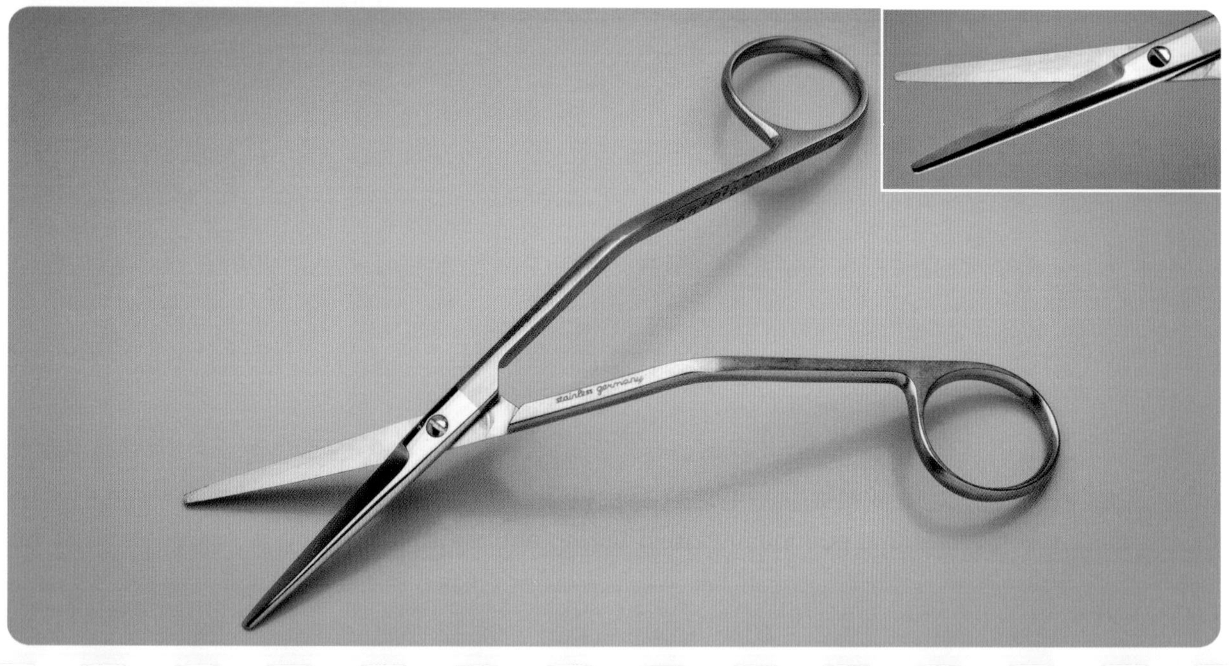

Scissors/Jansen

USE • To cut nasal septum cartilage

VARIETIES • Sharp or blunt angled blades

ALSO KNOWN AS • Knight angular scissors

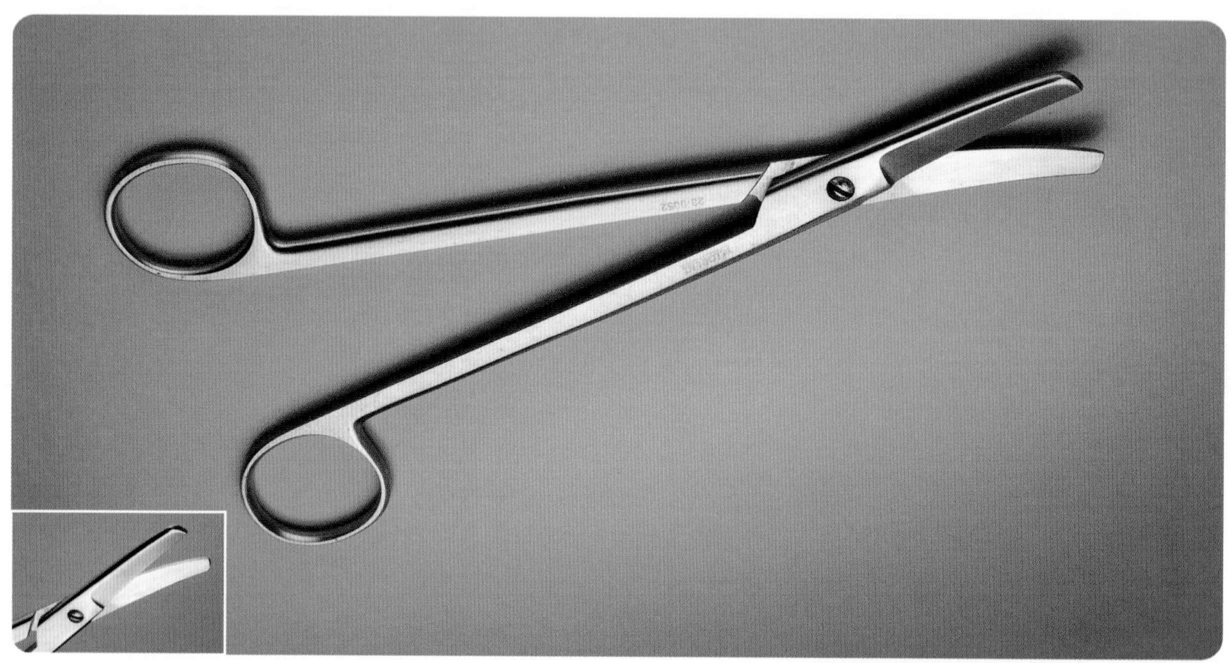

09

Scissors/Mayo

USE • To cut thick or tough tissue (e.g., fascia); to cut suture

VARIETIES • Straight or curved blades; various lengths

ALSO KNOWN AS • Doctor scissors, suture scissors

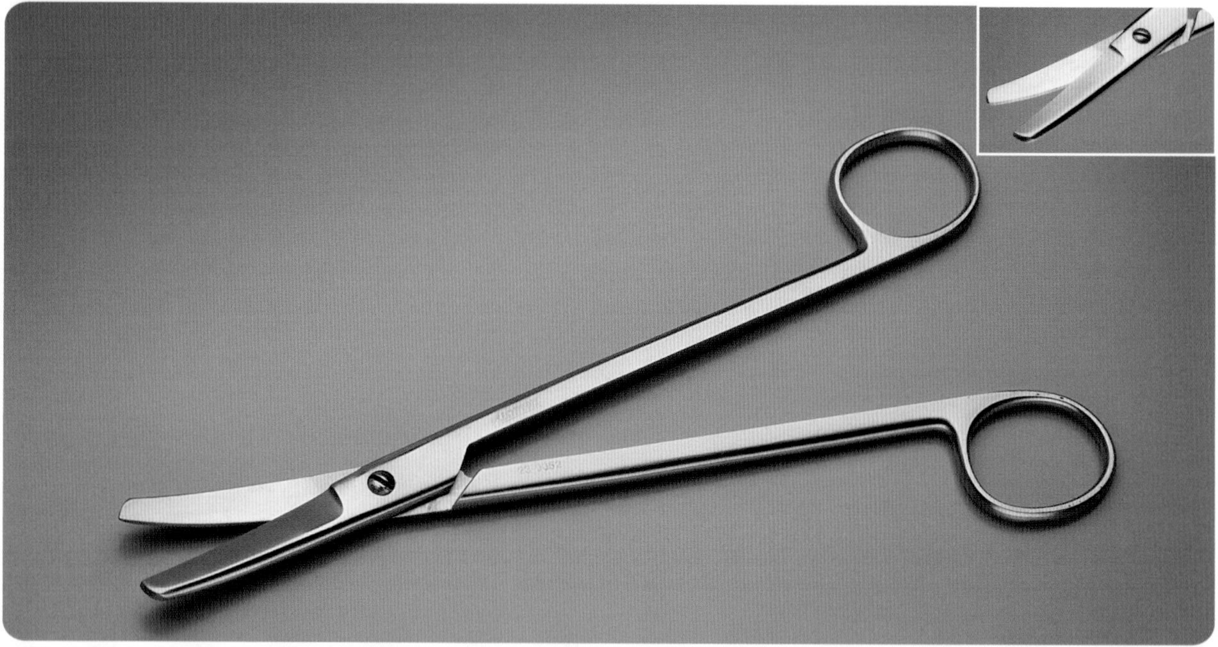

62

Scissors/Mayo-Sims

USE • To dissect tissue; to cut suture

VARIETIES • Straight or curved on flat blades; 7¾ inches long; sharp or blunt points

ALSO KNOWN AS • Deaver scissors, suture scissors

64

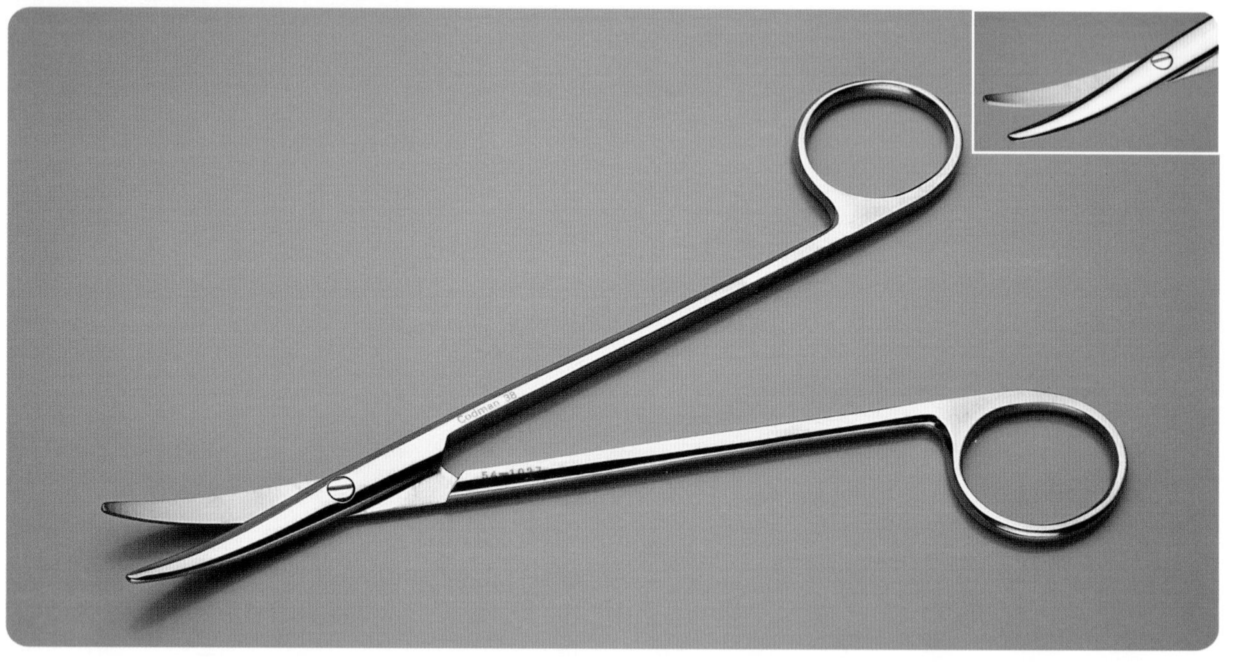

Scissors/Metzenbaum

USE • To dissect soft tissue

VARIETIES • Curved or straight on flat blades; various lengths

ALSO KNOWN AS • Metz, tissue scissors

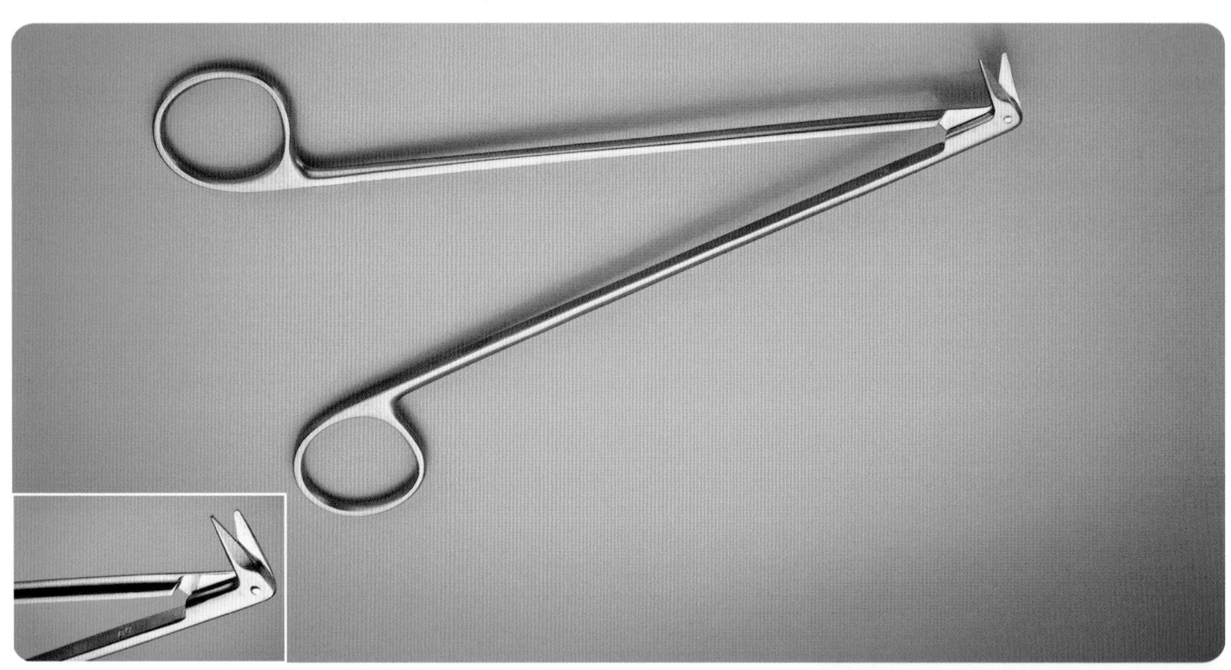

99

Scissors/Potts

USE • To extend venotomy or arteriotomy incisions

VARIETIES • 25 to 60 degree angled blades; various lengths; can be forward or reverse angles

ALSO KNOWN AS • Potts-Smith, vascular scissors

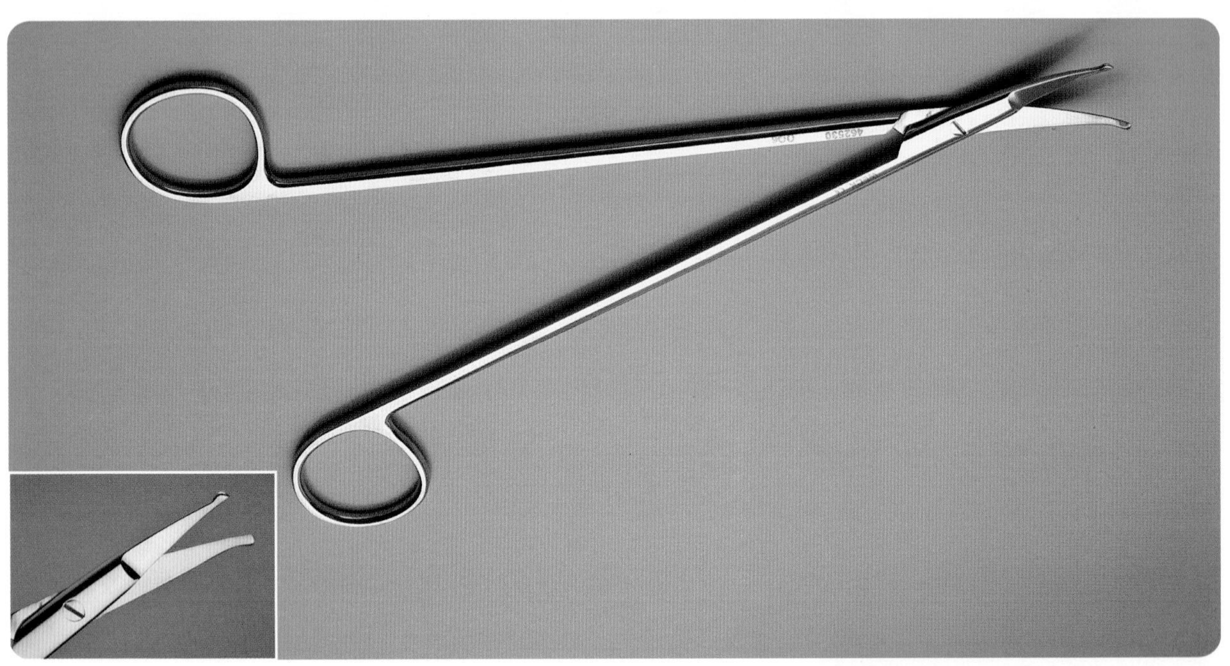

89

Scissors/Strully

USE • To cut fine tissue during abdominal surgery, neurosurgery, and vascular surgery

VARIETIES • Slightly curved blades with probe tips; 8 inches long

ALSO KNOWN AS • Dissecting scissors, neurological scissors

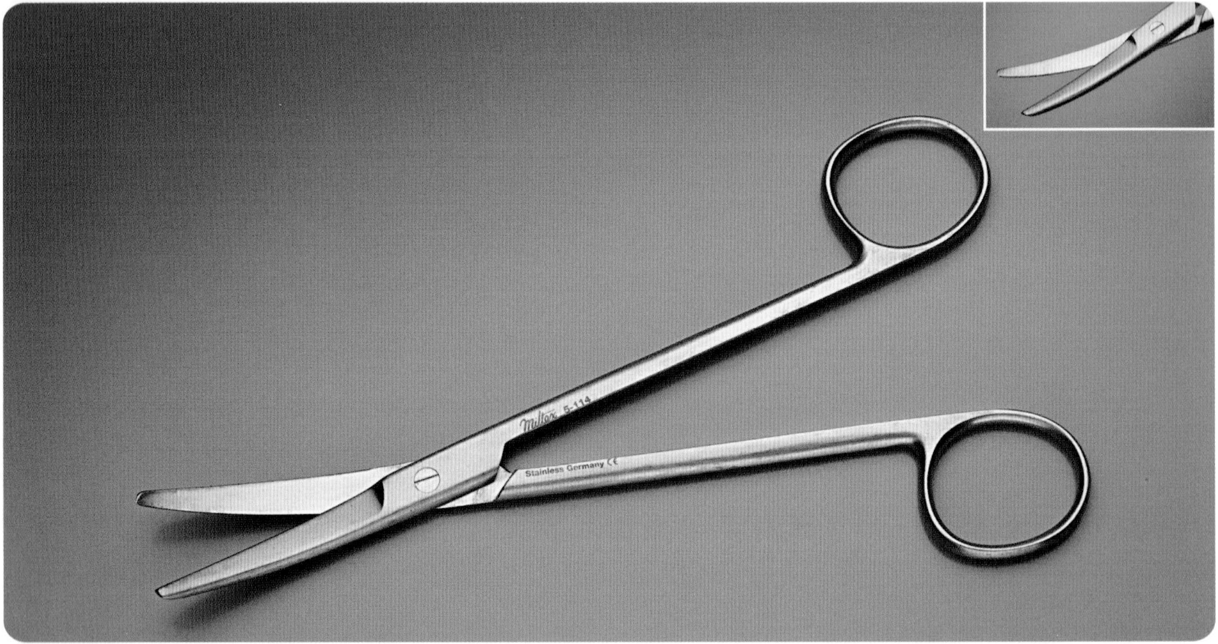
Miltex 5-114
Stainless Germany CE

Scissors/Suture

USE • To cut suture material

VARIETIES • Straight or curved; blunt/blunt or sharp/blunt blades; various lengths

ALSO KNOWN AS • Nurses scissors, operating scissors

72

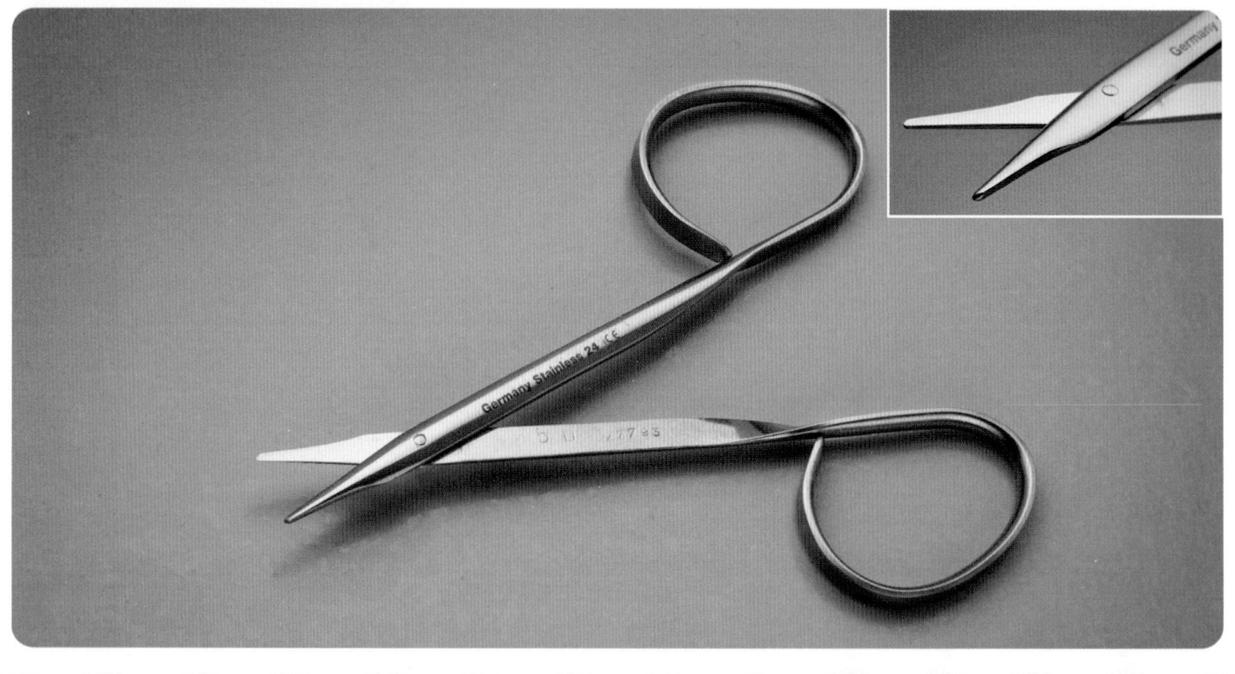

Scissors/Tenotomy

USE • To dissect fine tissue (e.g., in hand surgery); to penetrate tissue; to spread and cut tissue

VARIETIES • Short narrowed tip; straight or slightly curved blades; small size

ALSO KNOWN AS • Jameson Reynolds scissors, Stevens scissors

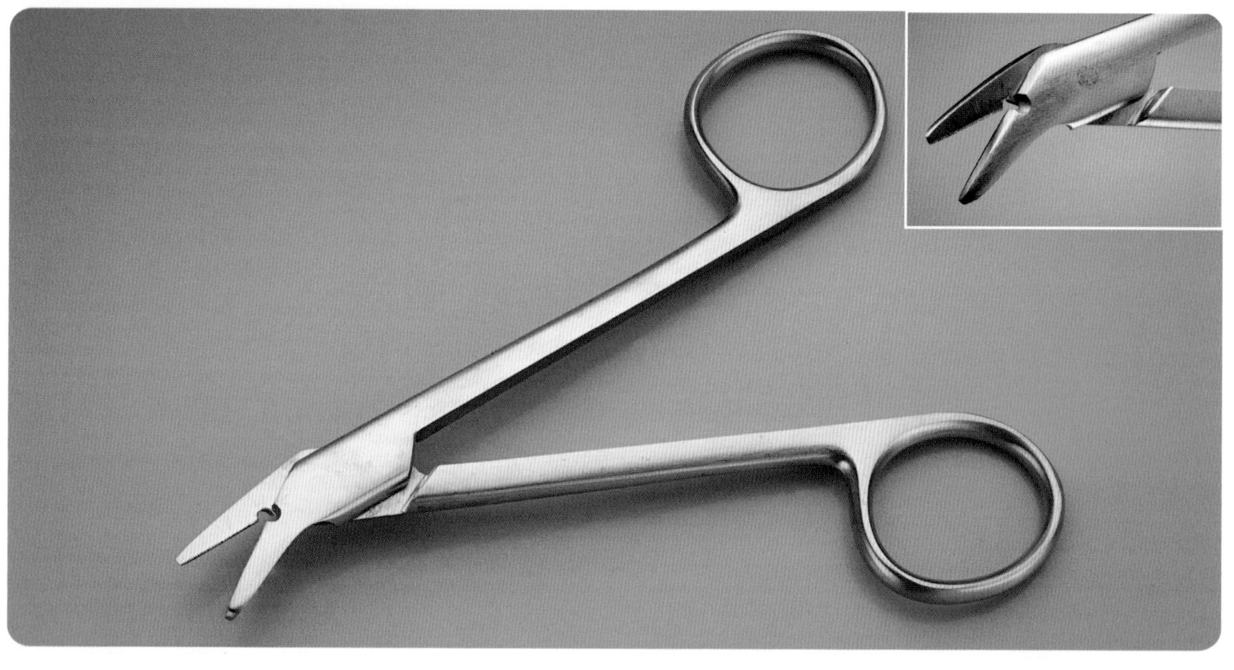

Scissors/Wire-Cutting

USE • To cut wire sutures

VARIETIES • Blades 4 3⁄4 inches long; angled to side; one serrated blade

ALSO KNOWN AS • Wire cutters

CHAPTER 2

Forceps/Grasping

Forceps are handheld hinged instruments used for grasping and holding objects. Forceps are used when fingers are too large to grasp small objects or when many objects need to be held at one time while the hands are used to perform a task.

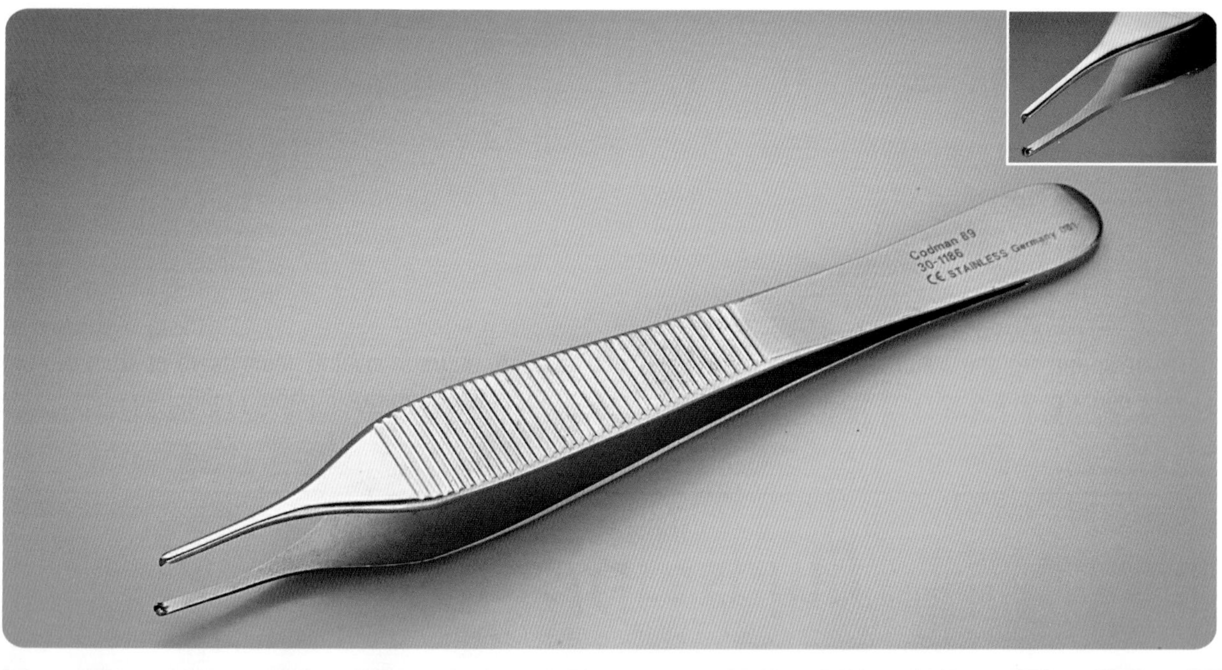
Codman 89
30-1186
CE STAINLESS Germany

Forceps/Adson

USE • To grasp superficial tissue (e.g., dermis)

VARIETIES • Smooth end or with 1 × 2 teeth or 2 × 3 teeth; 4¾ inches long

ALSO KNOWN AS • Bunny forceps, toothed Adson

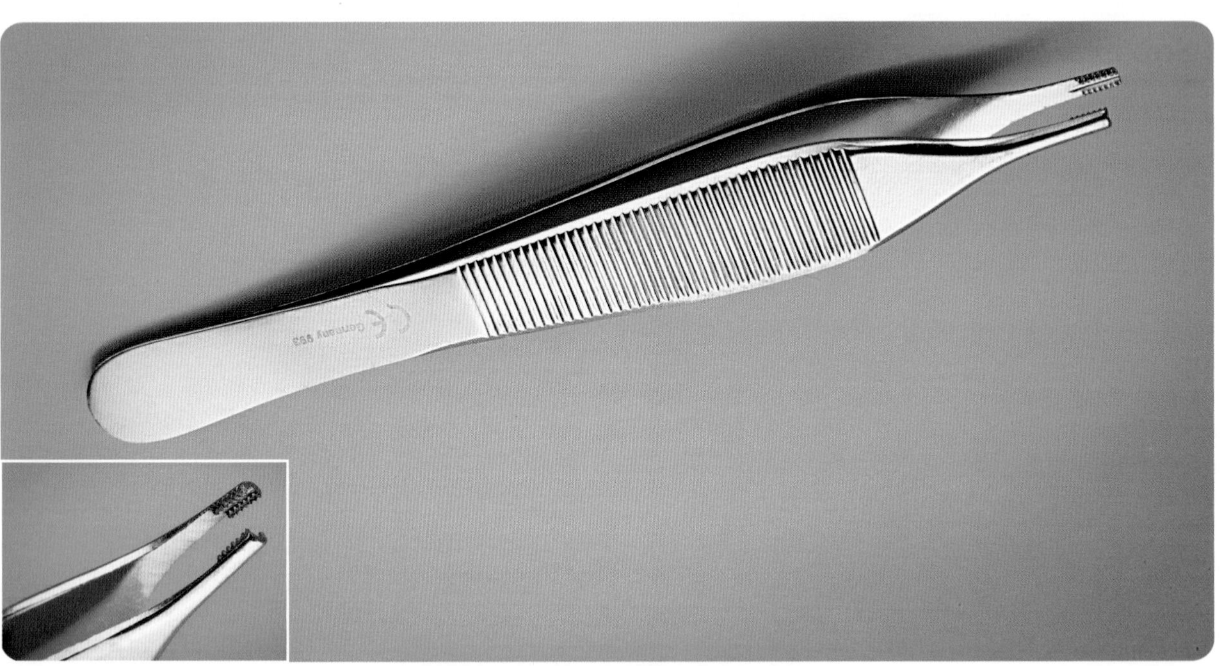

08

Forceps/Adson-Brown

USE • To grasp superficial, delicate tissue (e.g., during plastic surgery)

VARIETIES • 7 × 8 or 9 × 9 teeth; 4¾ inches long

ALSO KNOWN AS • Brown-Adson forceps

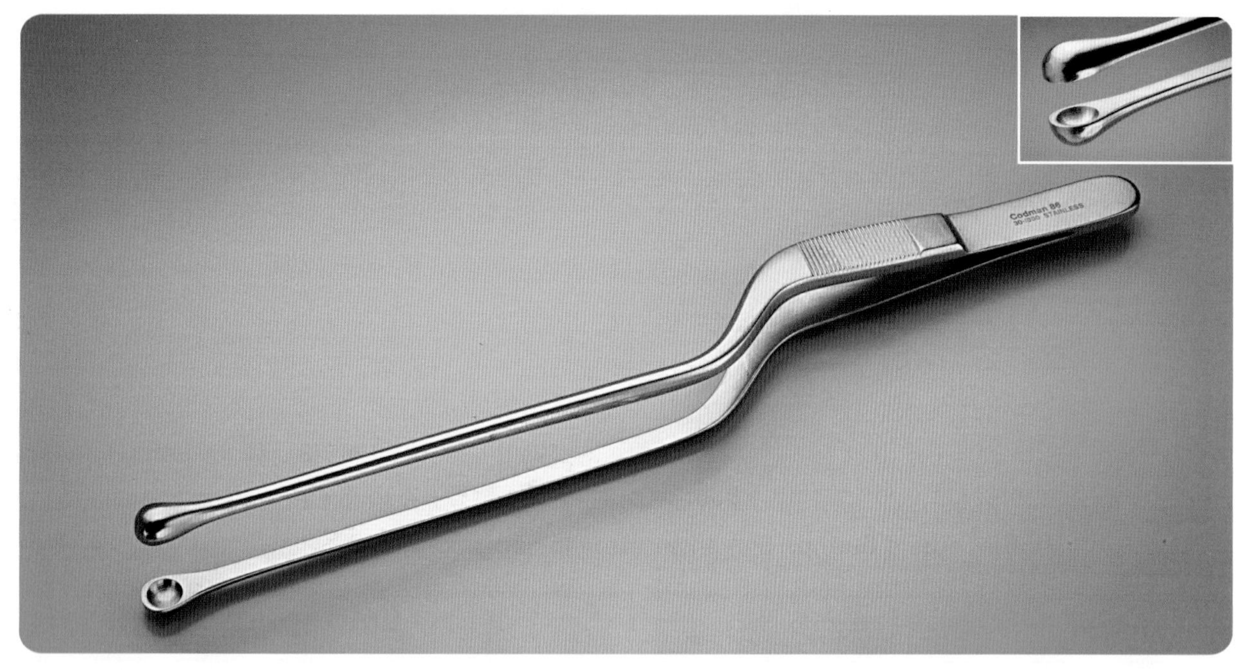
Codman 86
30-1830 STAINLESS

Forceps/Adson-Hypophyseal

USE • To grasp tissue during neurosurgery

VARIETIES • Bayonet-shaped; cupped jaws; 8¾ inches long

ALSO KNOWN AS • Bayonets, cup forceps

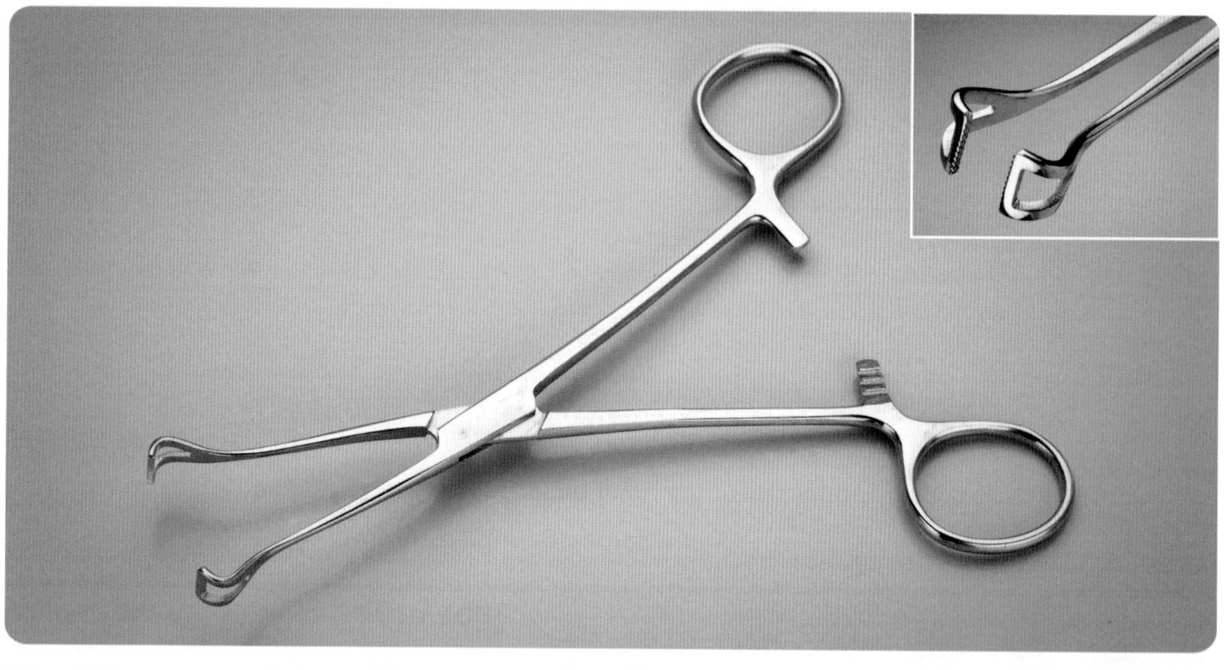

Forceps/Babcock

USE • To grasp delicate tissue (e.g., intestines, appendix) without crushing or traumatizing

VARIETIES • Heavy or delicate jaws; various lengths (5 ½ to 9 ½ inches)

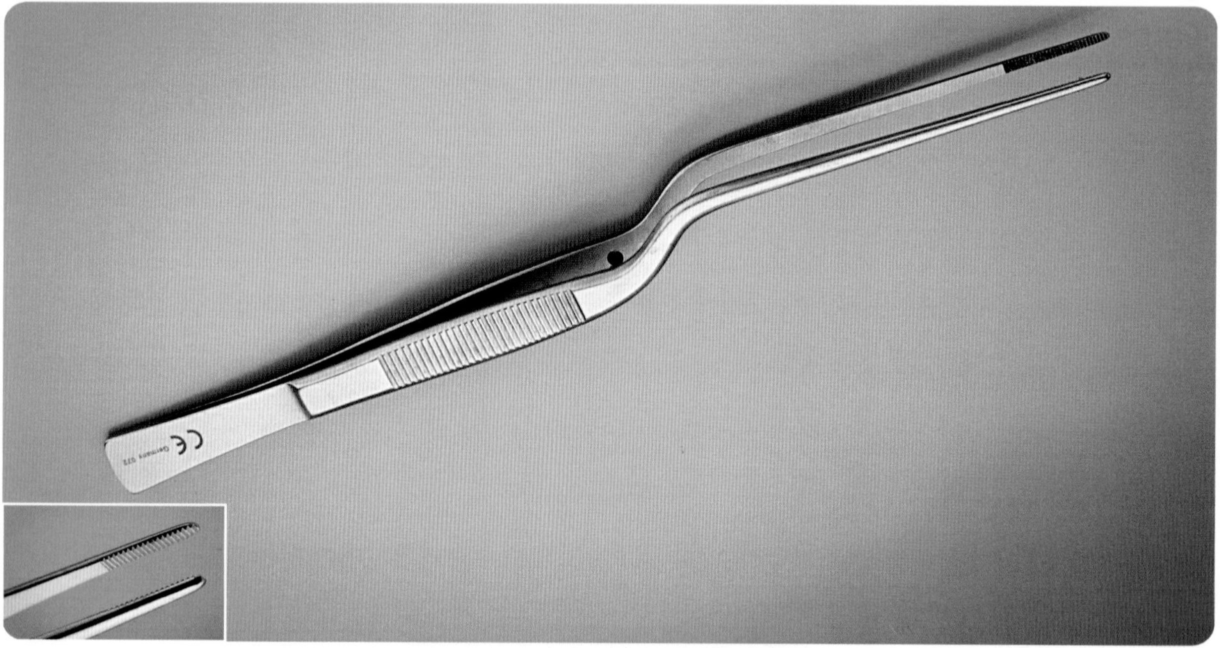

Forceps/Bayonet

USE • To grasp tissue during neurosurgery and some otorhinolaryngology (ear and nose) procedures

VARIETIES • Bayonet-shaped; can have serrated or 1 × 2 teeth; 6 ¼ to 8 inches long

ALSO KNOWN AS • Butler forceps, Cushing forceps

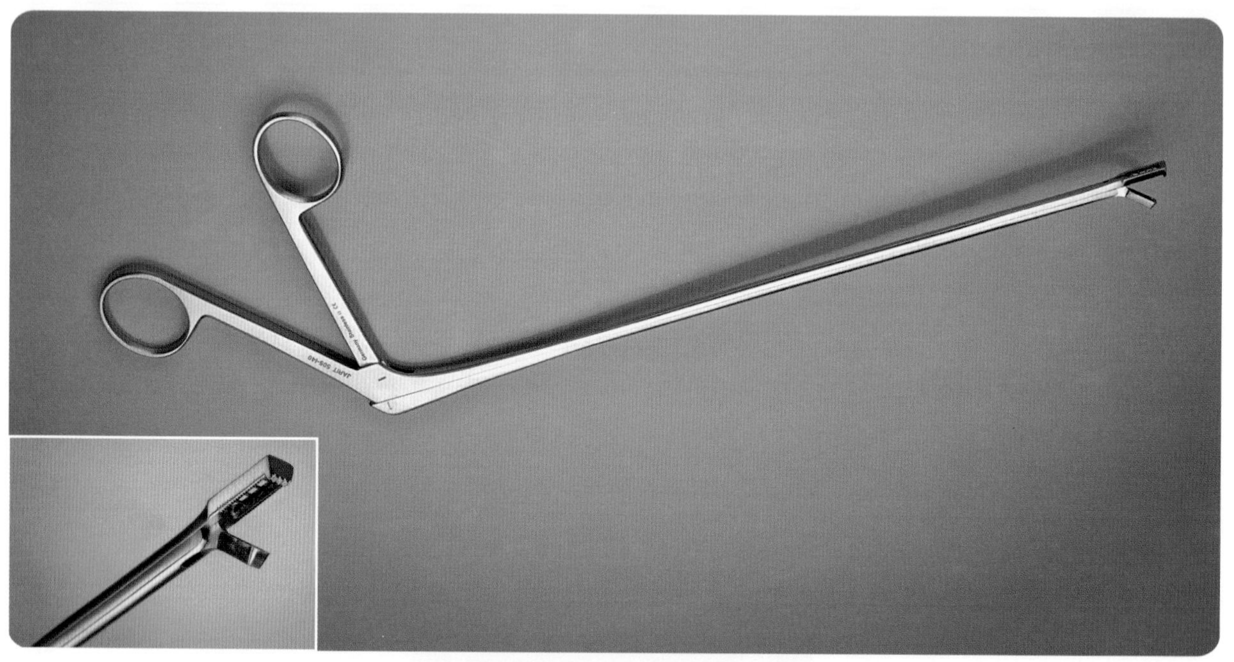

Forceps/Biopsy, Kevorkian

USE • To grasp tissue during transvaginal or transrectal tissue biopsy

VARIETIES • Sharp teeth; 10 inches long

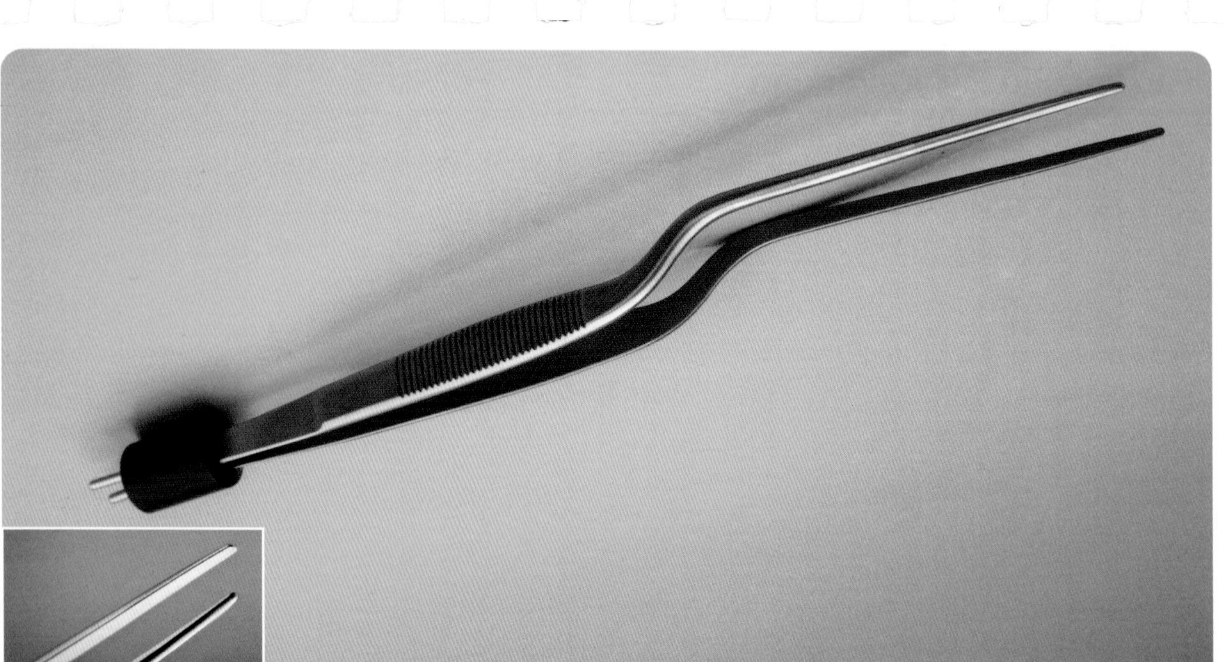

06

Forceps/Bipolar

USE • To grasp delicate tissue for electrosurgical coagulation (e.g., during neurosurgery or infertility surgical procedures)

VARIETIES • Bayonet-shaped or straight; fine-point tips

ALSO KNOWN AS • Jeweler's forceps, microtip forceps, rhoton forceps

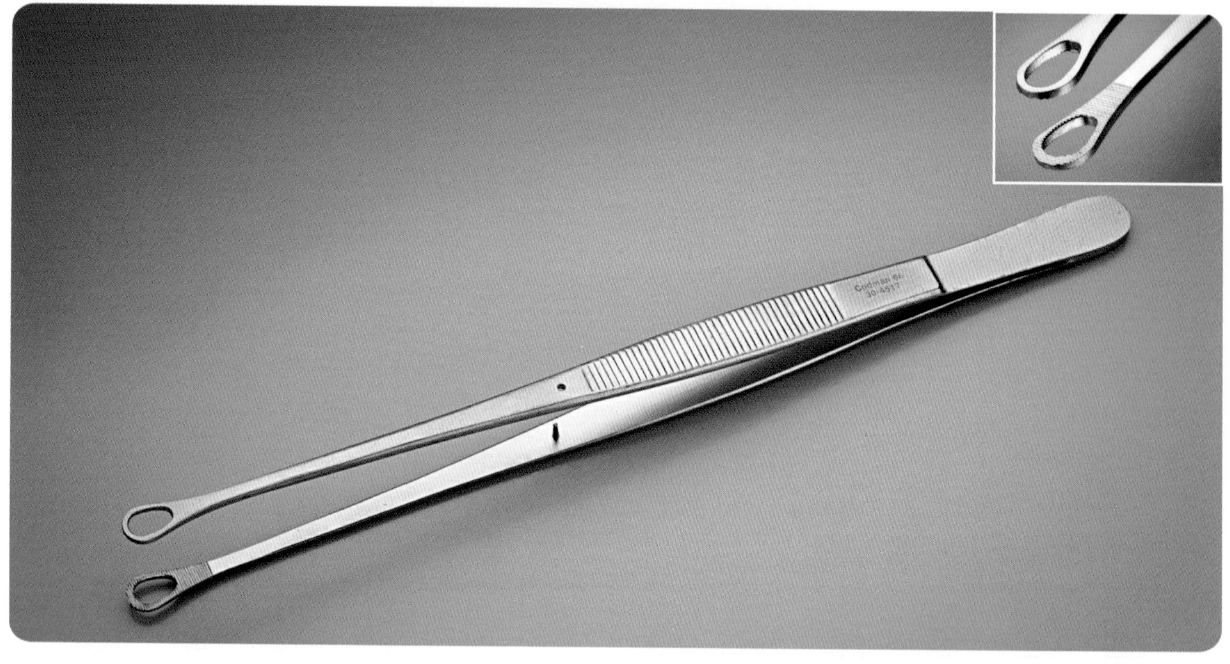
Codman 66
30-4517

Forceps/Brain Tissue

USE • To grasp delicate brain tissue during neurosurgery

VARIETIES • Cup or ring tips

ALSO KNOWN AS • Ring forceps

94

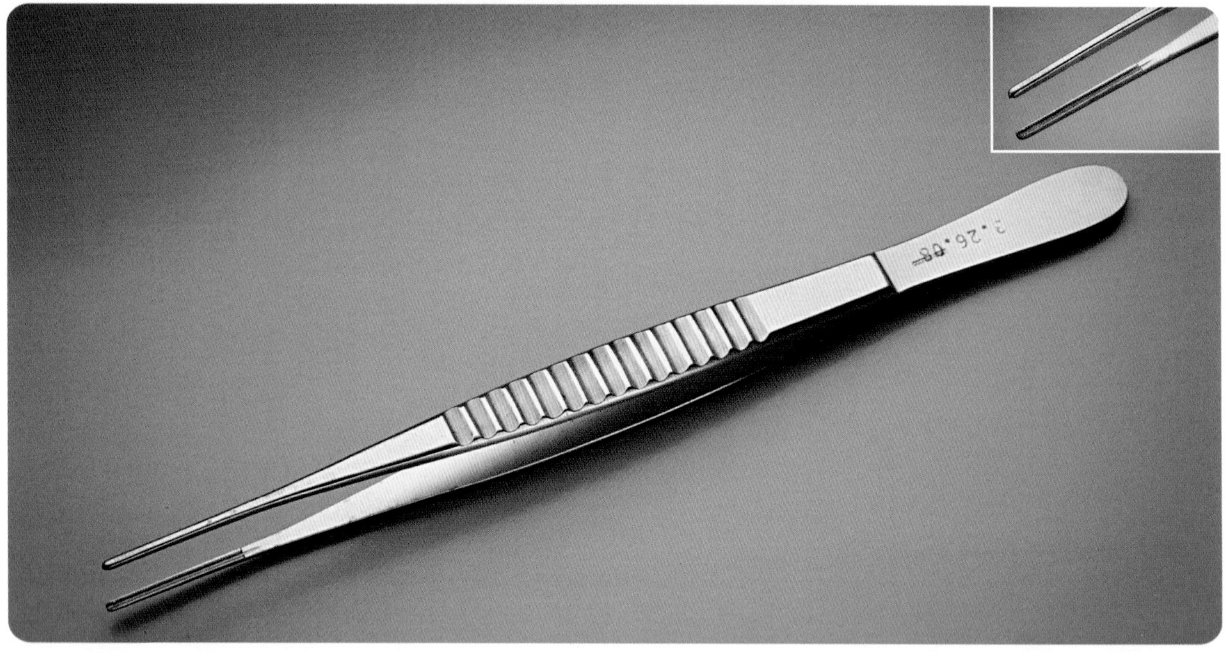

Forceps/DeBakey

USE • To grasp fine or heavy tissue (e.g., during vascular or cardiovascular surgery)

VARIETIES • Straight or angled tip; various tip lengths; various jaw tip widths

ALSO KNOWN AS • DeBakey thoracic tissue forceps, DeBakey vascular tissue forceps

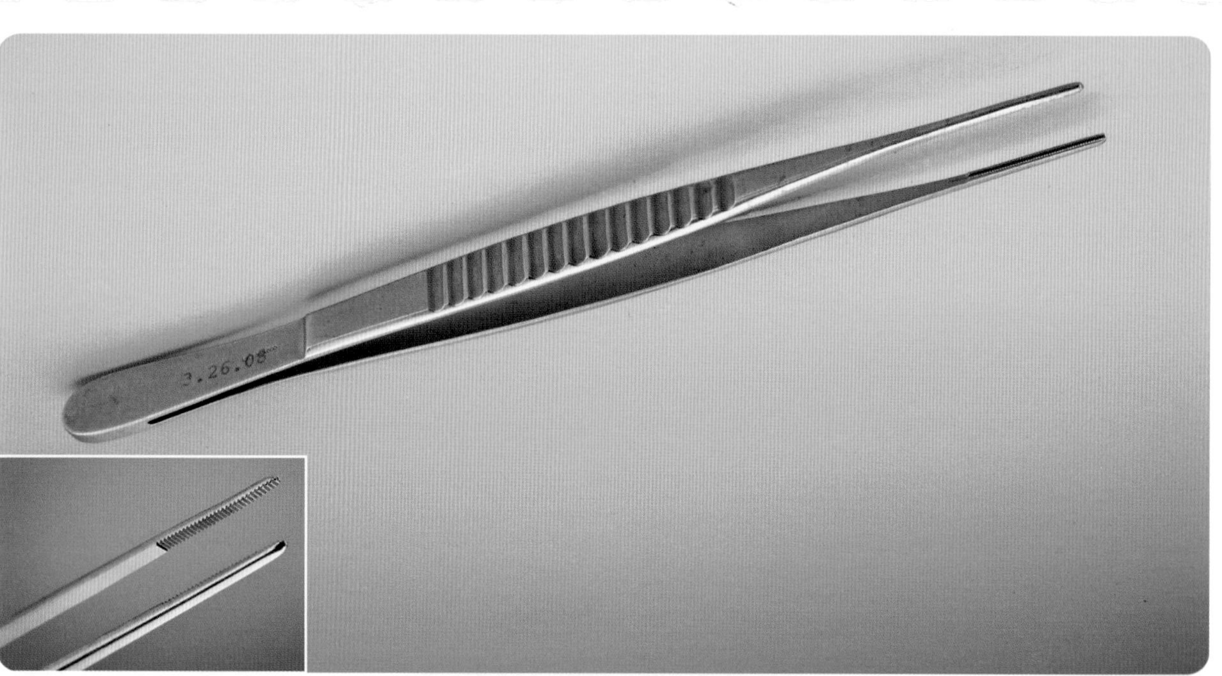
3.26.08

Forceps/Dressing

USE • To pick up or grasp tissue or items in the surgical wound to use for wound dressing and packing

VARIETIES • Delicate to heavy; various lengths

ALSO KNOWN AS • Packing forceps, pick ups, plain forceps

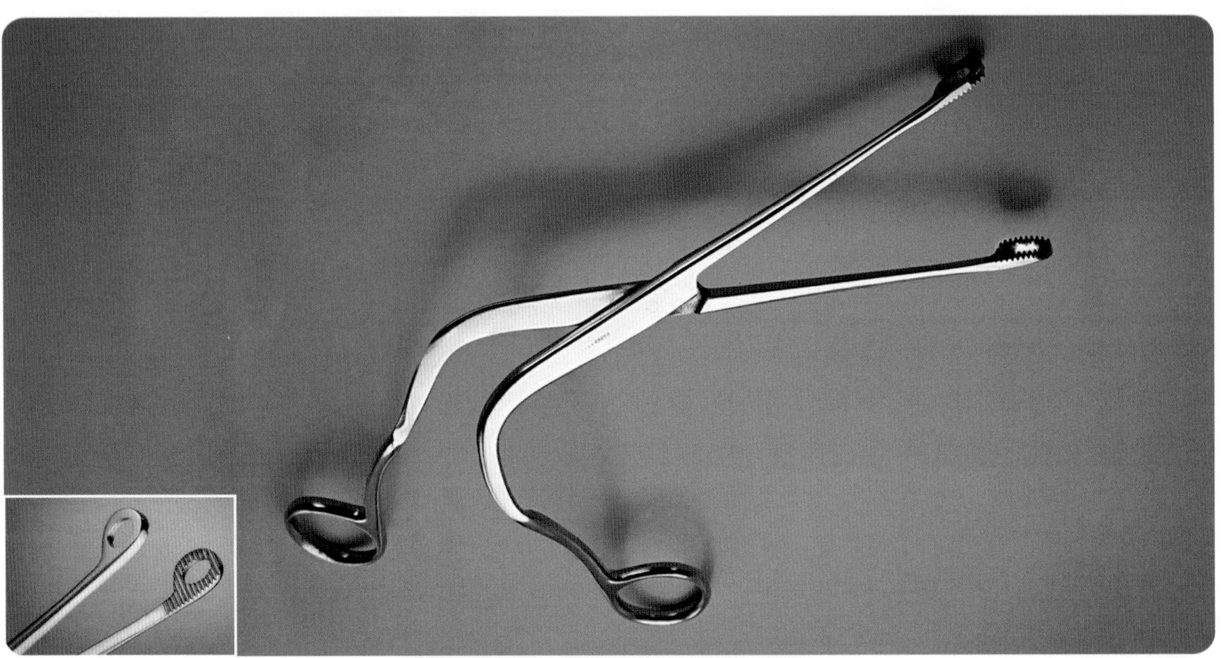

Forceps/Endotracheal, Magill

USE • To hold cotton balls to swab the vocal cords before intubation

VARIETIES • Open or closed jaw; pediatric and adult sizes

ALSO KNOWN AS • Intubating forceps

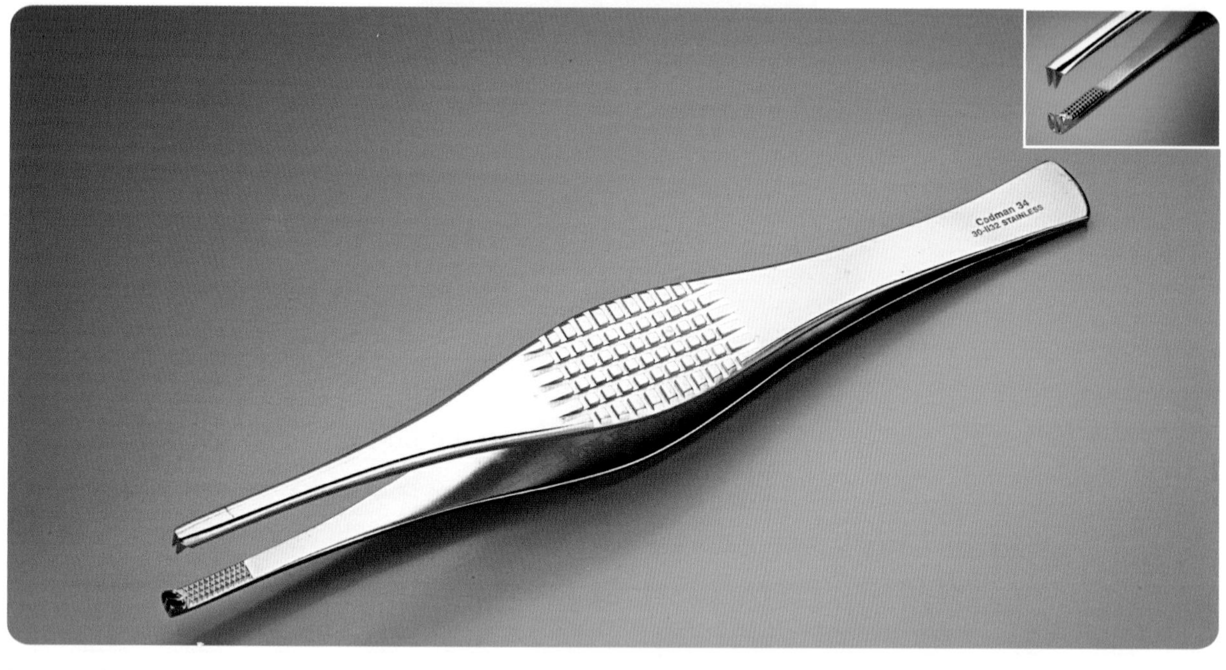
Codman 34
30-1132 STAINLESS

Forceps/Ferris Smith

USE • To grasp tissue during orthopedic procedures; to close fascia

VARIETIES • Heavy; 1 × 2 teeth or 2 × 3 teeth; 6¾ inches long

ALSO KNOWN AS • Bonnie forceps

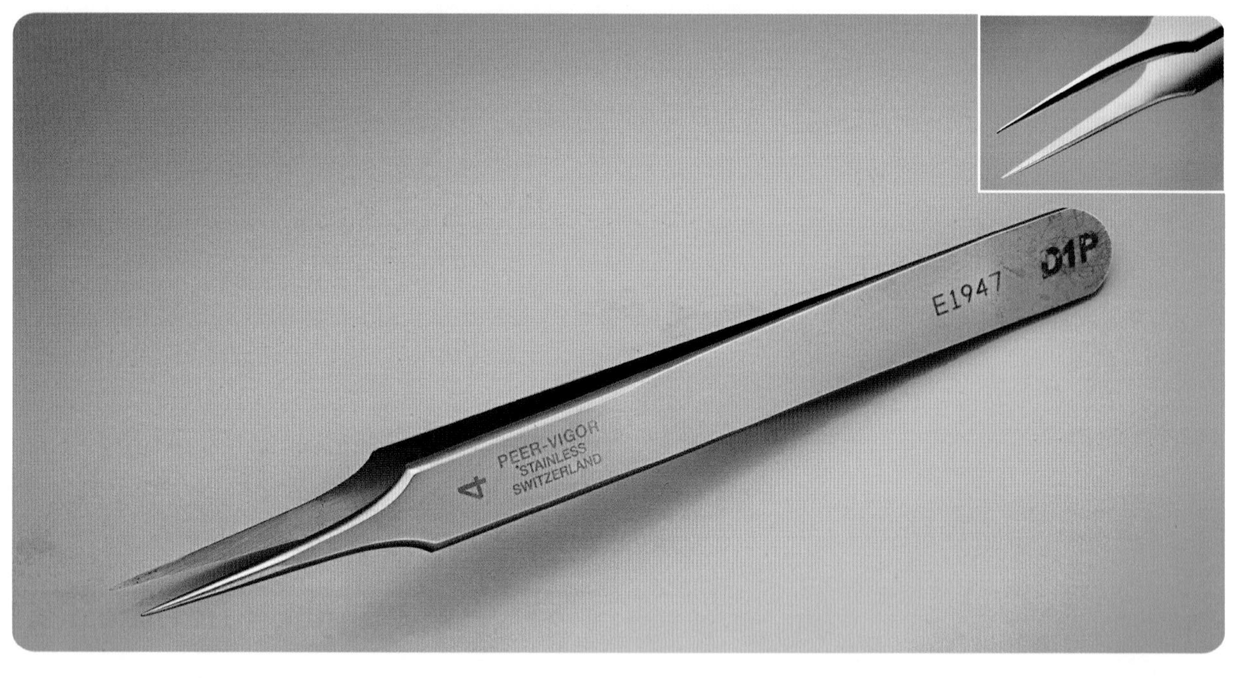
4
PEER-VIGOR
'STAINLESS
SWITZERLAND
E1947
01P

Forceps/Jeweler's

USE • To grasp fine tissue during ophthalmic and microvascular hand surgery

VARIETIES • Straight or curved tips; short or long lengths

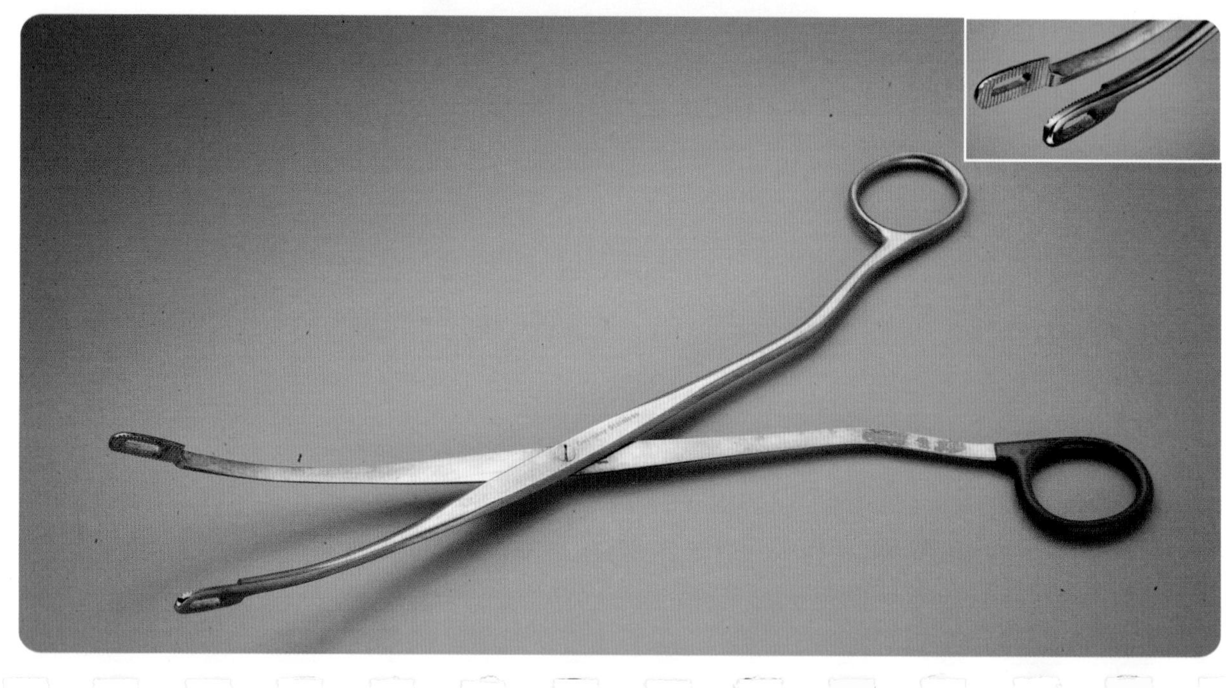

Forceps/Kidney Stone

USE • To grasp renal calculi or polyps

VARIETIES • Ring handled; quarter curved, half curved, three-quarter curved, or fully curved jaws; 9 ½ inches long

ALSO KNOWN AS • Mazzariello-Caprini forceps, Randall forceps

106

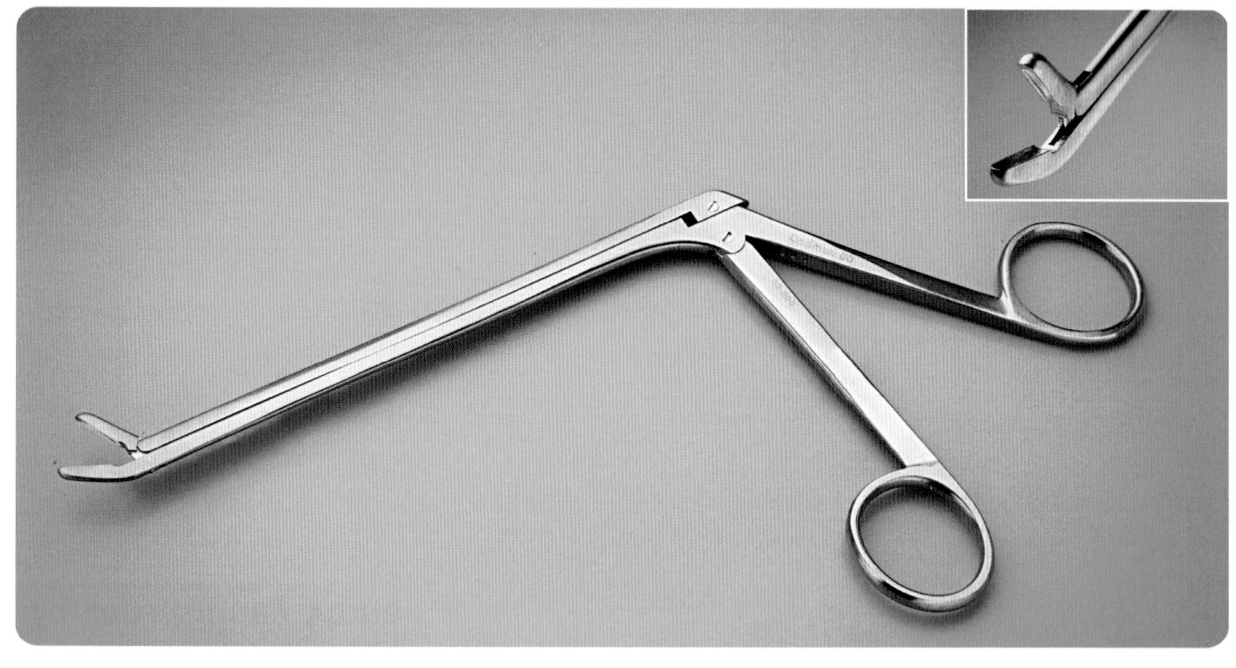

Forceps/Nasal

USE • To grasp or cut tissue during intranasal surgery (e.g., rhinoplasty, submucous resection, nasal polypectomy)

VARIETIES • Cutting or noncutting; alligator style; heavy or fine jaws; 5 to 7 inches long

ALSO KNOWN AS • Hartmann forceps, Knight forceps, Noyes forceps

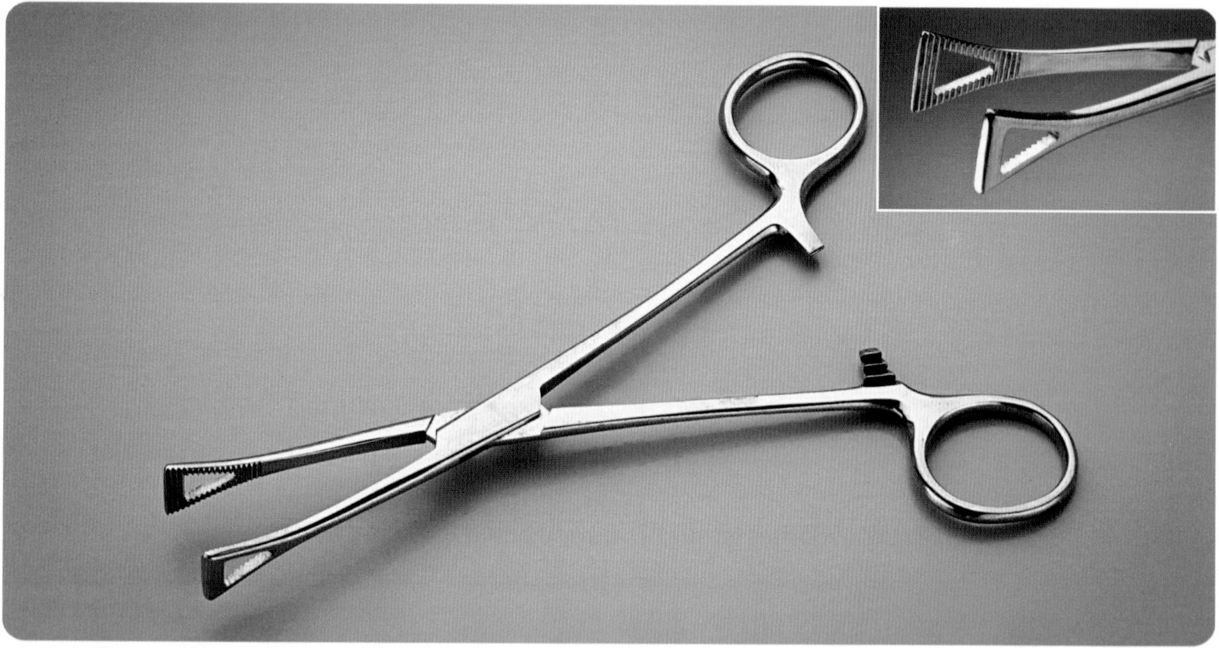

Forceps/Pennington

USE • To grasp tissue and organs during general surgery, especially rectal procedures

VARIETIES • Triangular jaws; 6 to 8 inches long

ALSO KNOWN AS • Pennington tissue grasping forceps

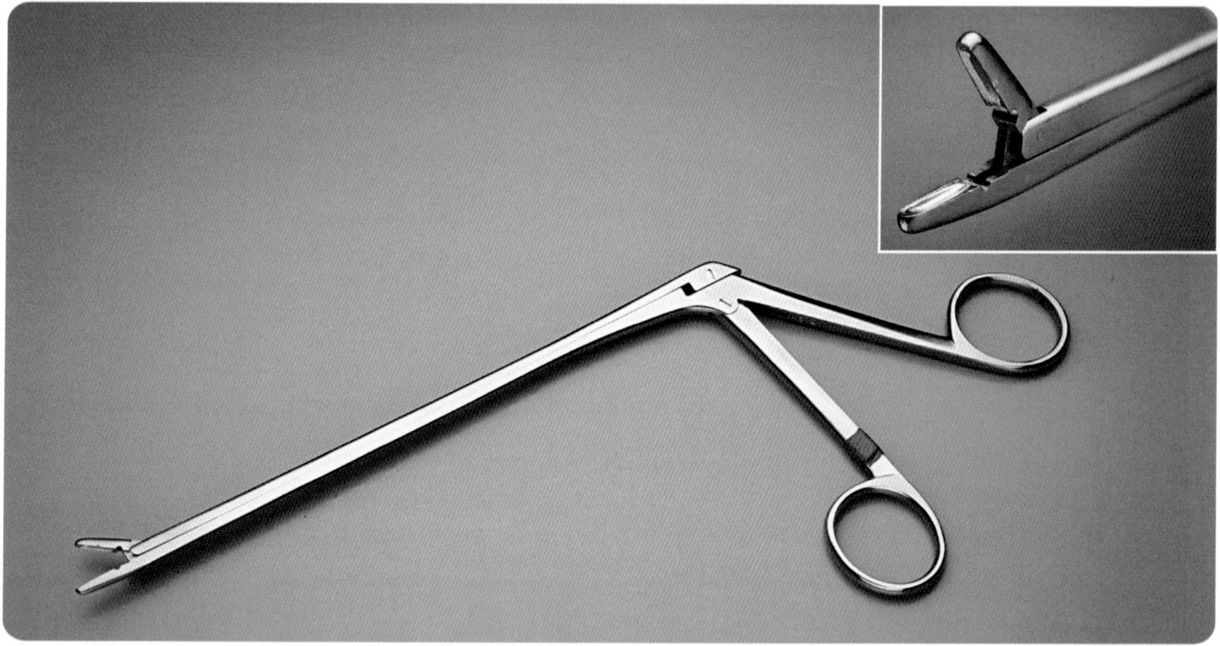

Forceps/Pituitary

USE • To grasp tissue during neurosurgical procedures (e.g., laminectomy)

VARIETIES • Up bite, down bite, or straight; 2 × 10 mm to 4 × 10 mm cups; 5 to 7 inches long

ALSO KNOWN AS • Love-Gruenwald forceps, Spurling forceps, Wilde forceps

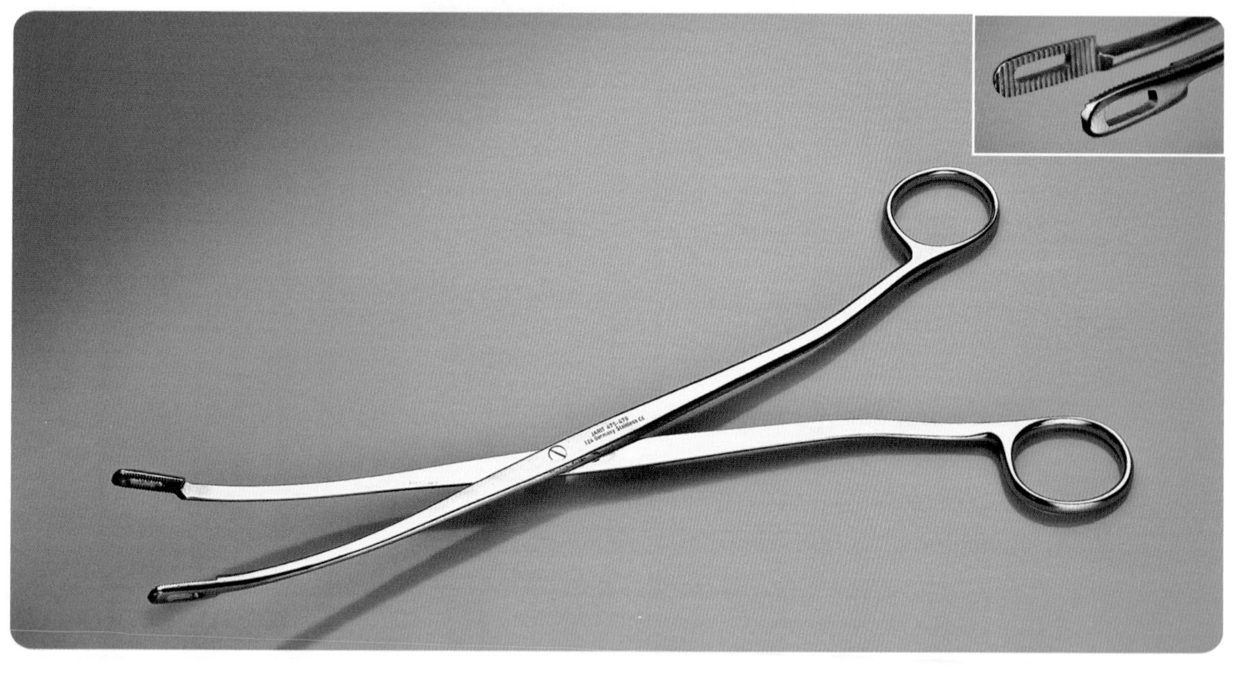

Forceps/Polyp

USE • Intrauterine: To grasp cervical polyps or intrauterine polyps

Gallbladder tissue: To grasp gallstones

VARIETIES • Small or large tips; straight or curved

ALSO KNOWN AS • Desjardins gallstone forceps

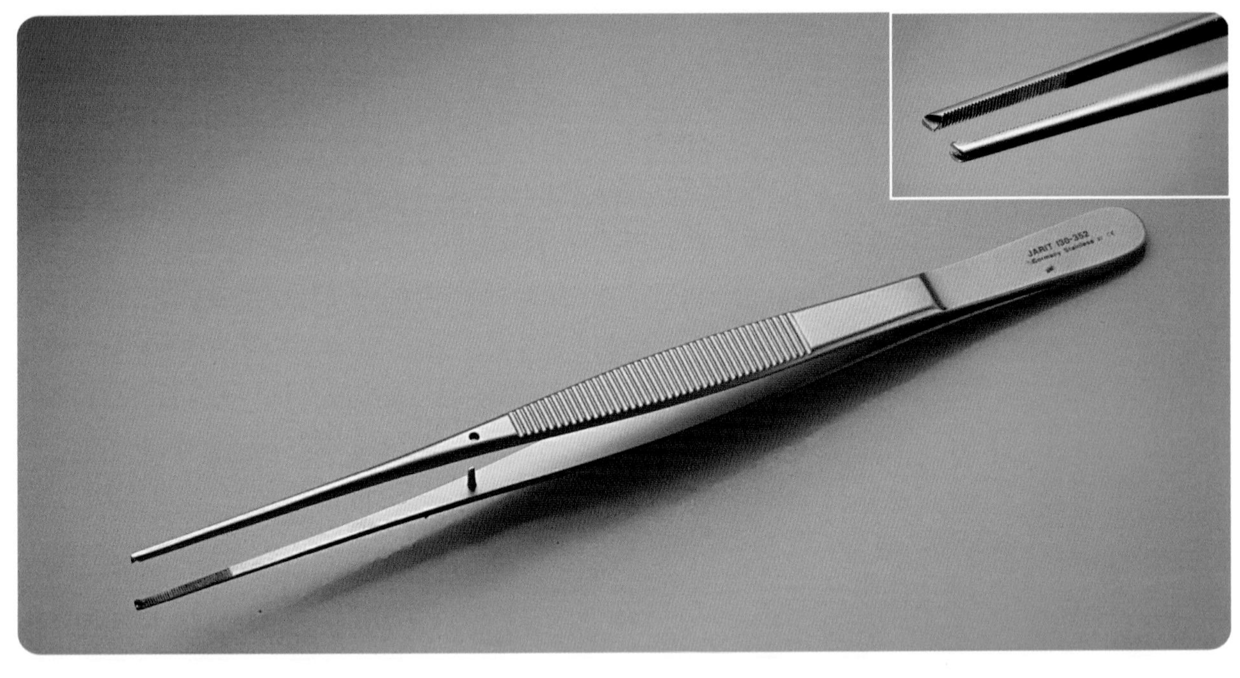
JARIT 130-352

Forceps/Potts-Smith

USE • To grasp tissue during vascular (particularly neurovascular) surgery

VARIETIES • 1 × 2 teeth or serrated tip; various lengths

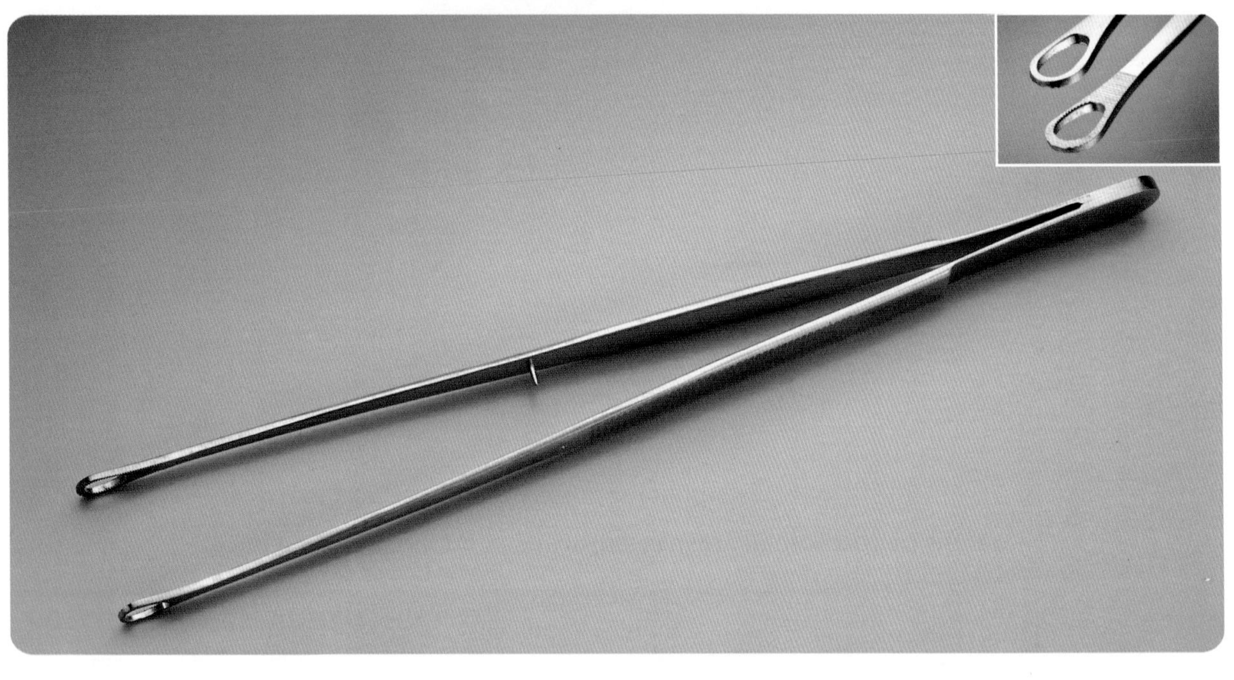

Forceps/Ring

USE • To hold sponges while prepping; for deep, blunt dissection of soft tissue

VARIETIES • Various lengths

ALSO KNOWN AS • Singley forceps

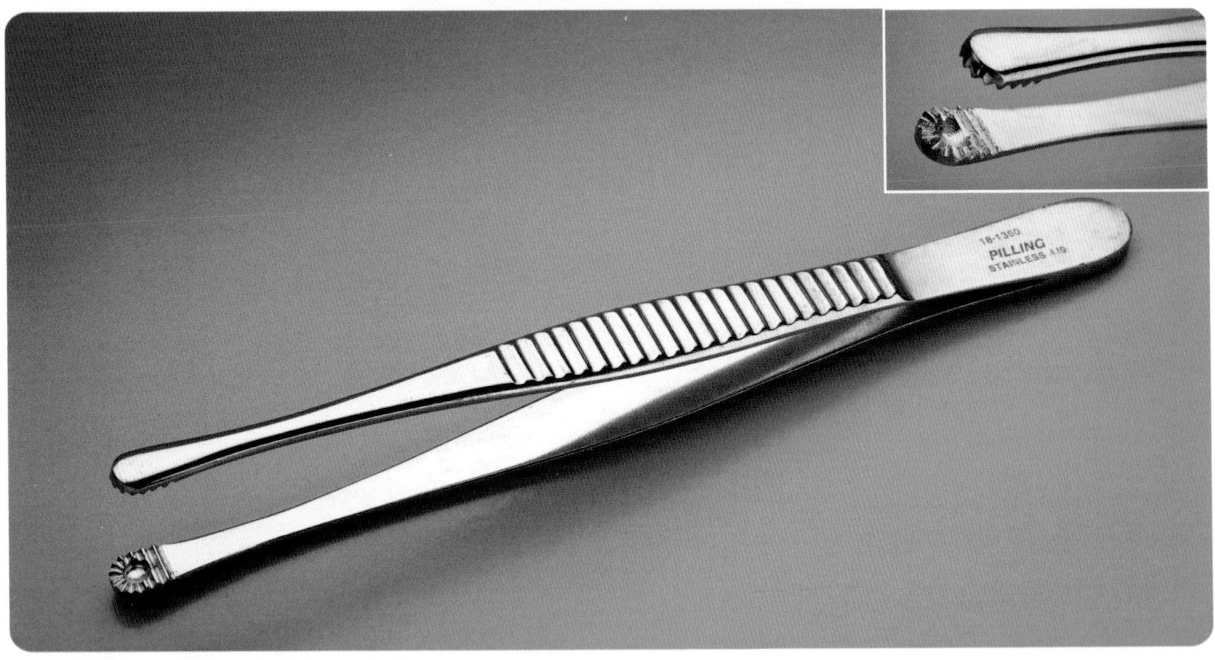
18-1350
PILLING
STAINLESS

Forceps/Russian

USE • To approximate tissue during wound closure (e.g., abdominal wall fascia, uterus); to lift clots when evacuating hematomas

VARIETIES • 6, 8, or 10 inches long

120

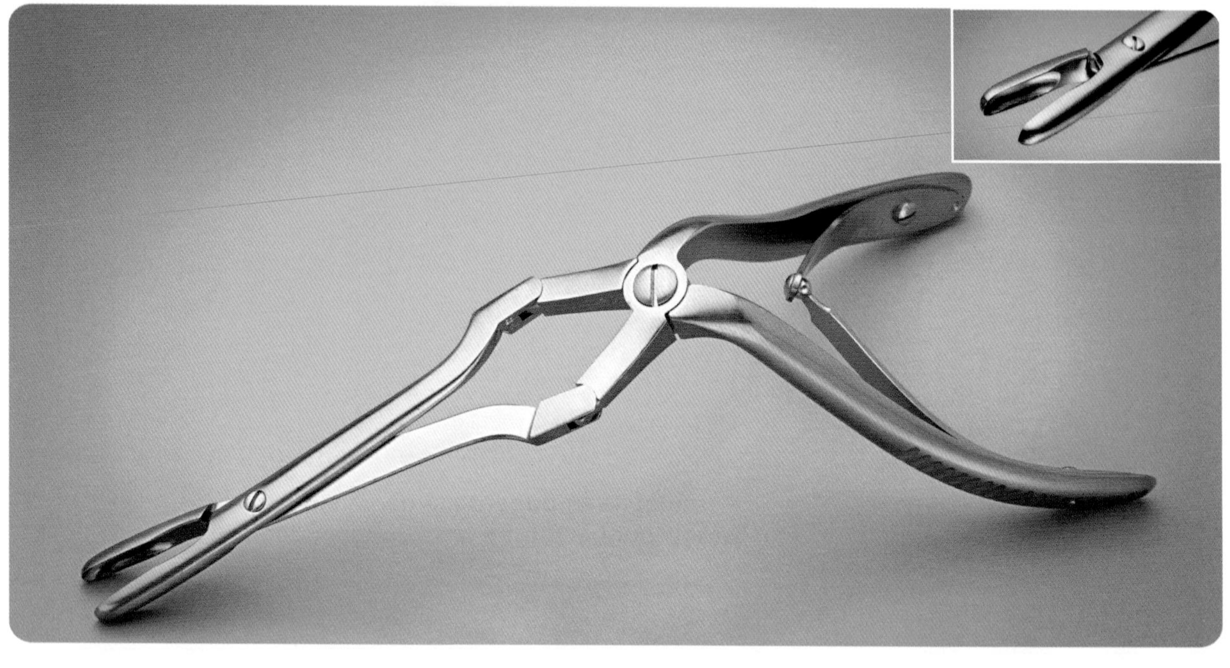

Forceps/Septum, Jansen

USE • To grasp the septum during nasal or plastic surgery

VARIETIES • Double action, spoon-shaped blades

ALSO KNOWN AS • Jansen-Middleton forceps

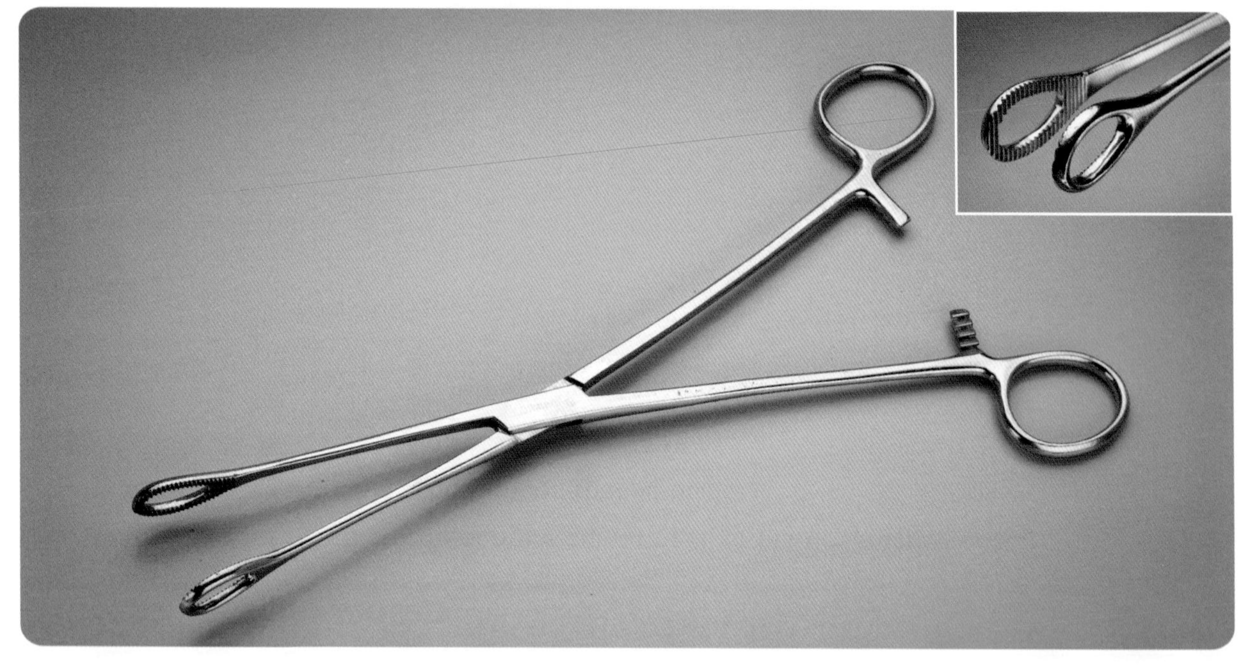

Forceps/Sponge

USE • To hold a sponge during patient's preoperative skin prep or intraoperative hemostatic exposure

VARIETIES • Straight or curved blades; long or short; smooth or serrated jaws

ALSO KNOWN AS • Fletcher sponge forceps, Foerster sponge forceps, ring forceps, sponge stick

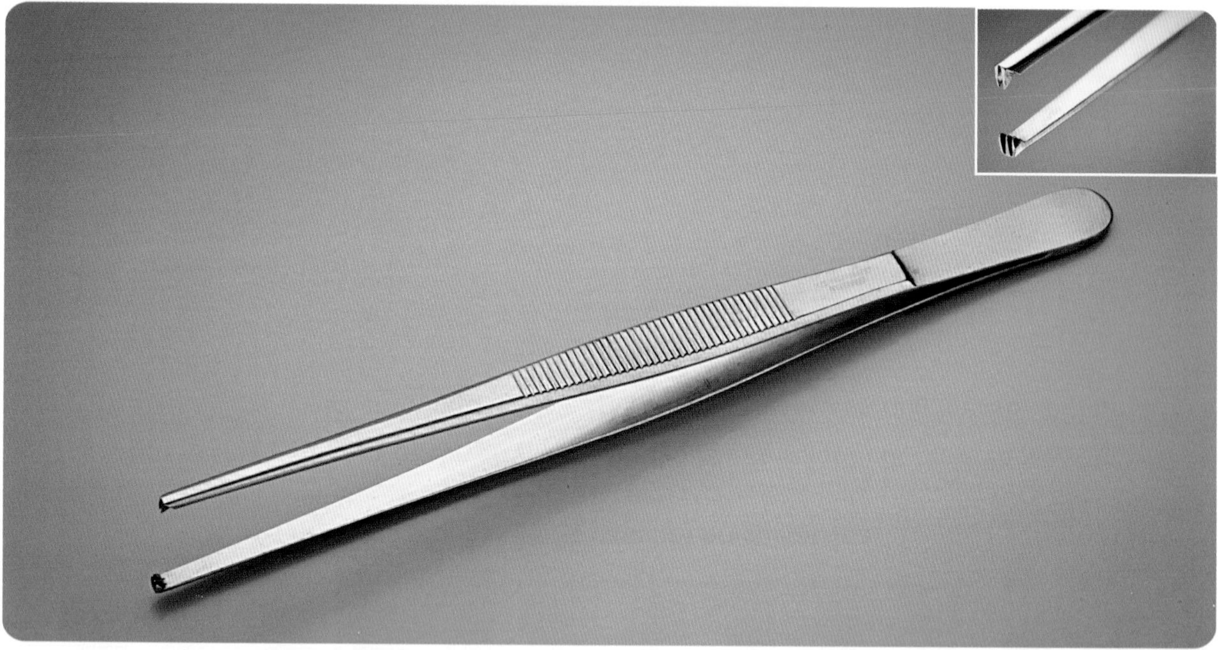

124

Forceps/Tissue

USE • To grasp or pick up soft tissue or bony tissue

VARIETIES • 1 × 2, 2 × 3, 3 × 4, or 4 × 5 teeth; various lengths

ALSO KNOWN AS • Toothed forceps, toothed tissue forceps

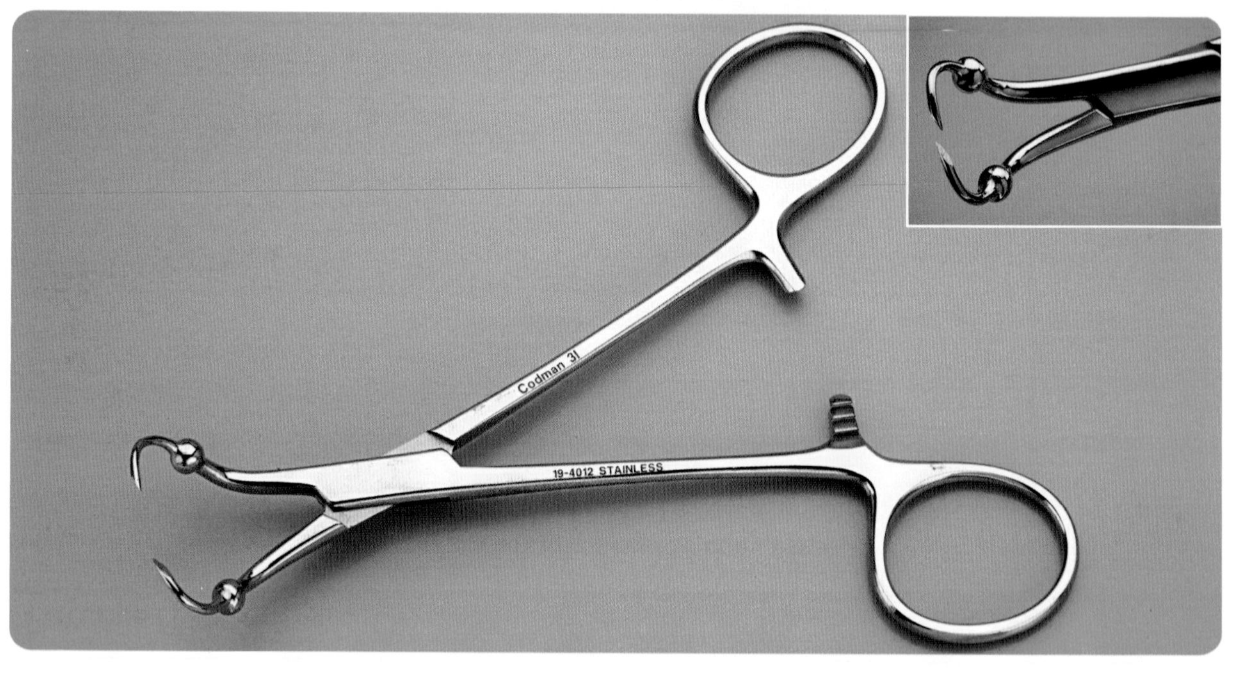
Codman 31
19-4012 STAINLESS

Forceps/Towel

USE • To attach and secure drape material; to grasp tissue for the purpose of applying traction or bone reduction for a fracture

VARIETIES • Perforating or nonperforating; hinged or spring activated; with or without ballstops; various lengths; blunt or sharp

ALSO KNOWN AS • Backhaus forceps, bone holder, Edna forceps, Jones forceps, Peers forceps, Roeder towel clamp, towel clip

CHAPTER 3

Clamps/Holding

Clamps are devices used to hold objects in fixed positions. They are occluders for blood vessels and other organs.

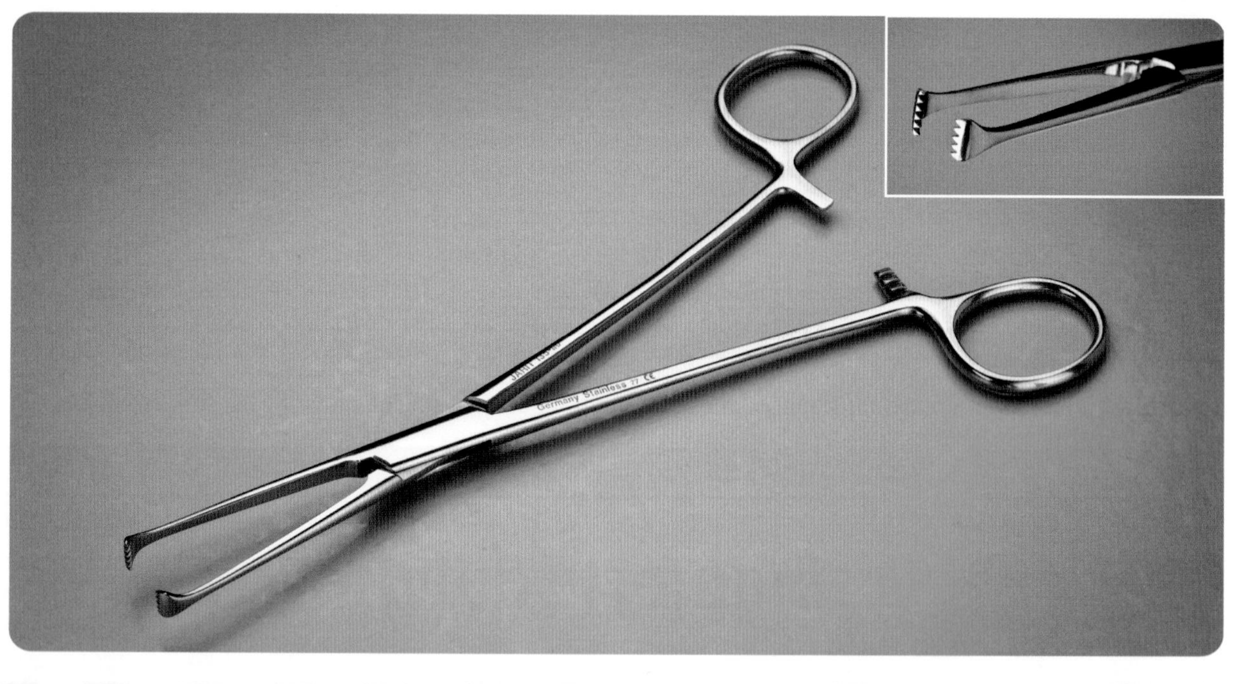

Clamp/Allis

USE • To grasp and hold tissues or organs; to secure any operating material (e.g., cords and suction tubing) onto the drapes

VARIETIES • 4 × 5, 5 × 6, or 9 × 10 teeth; various lengths; angular jaws

132

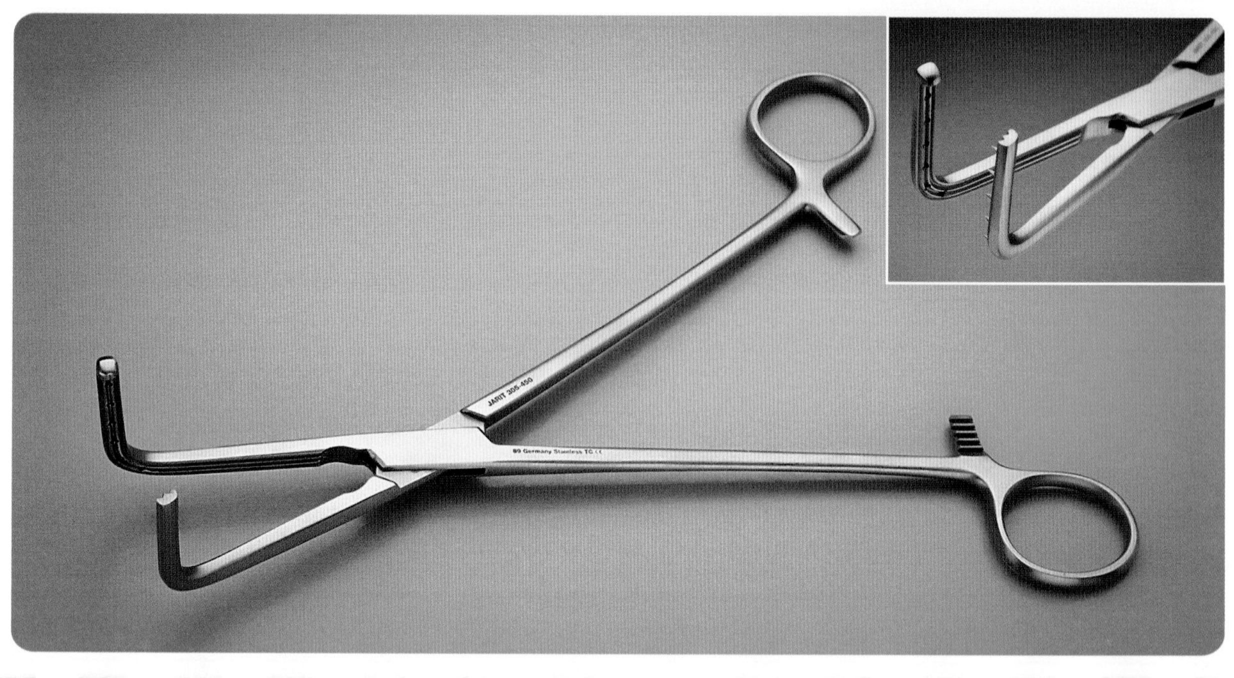

Clamp/Bronchus

USE • To secure a part of the lung during pulmonary surgery

VARIETIES • Angled; atraumatic teeth

ALSO KNOWN AS • Cooley clamp, Lees clamp, Sarot clamp

134

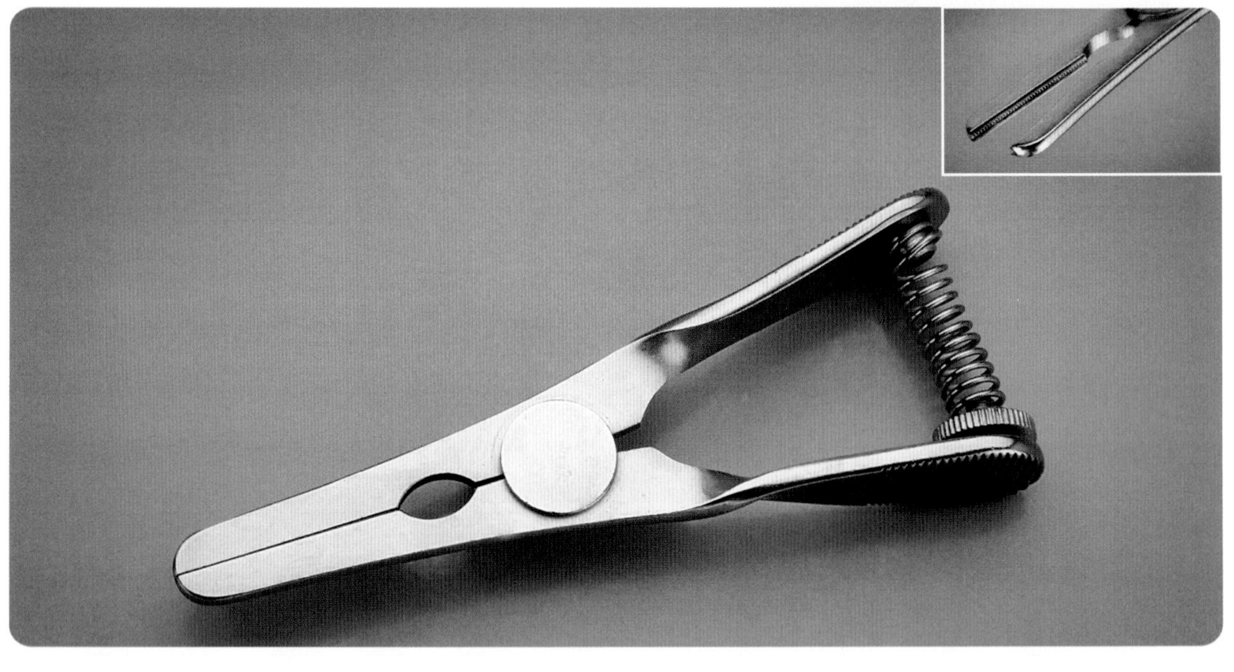

Clamp/Bulldog

USE • To occlude an artery or vein with correct tension to produce minimal trauma to vessels; clamps have low closing pressure for noncompressive occlusion (e.g., for coronary artery bypass or arteriovenous fistula)

VARIETIES • 2 to 6 cm jaw lengths; various overall lengths; straight or curved; disposable

ALSO KNOWN AS • Cooley bulldog clamp, DeBakey ring-handled bulldog clamp, Gregory soft bulldog clamp, microbulldog clamp, Wickham bulldog clamp

136

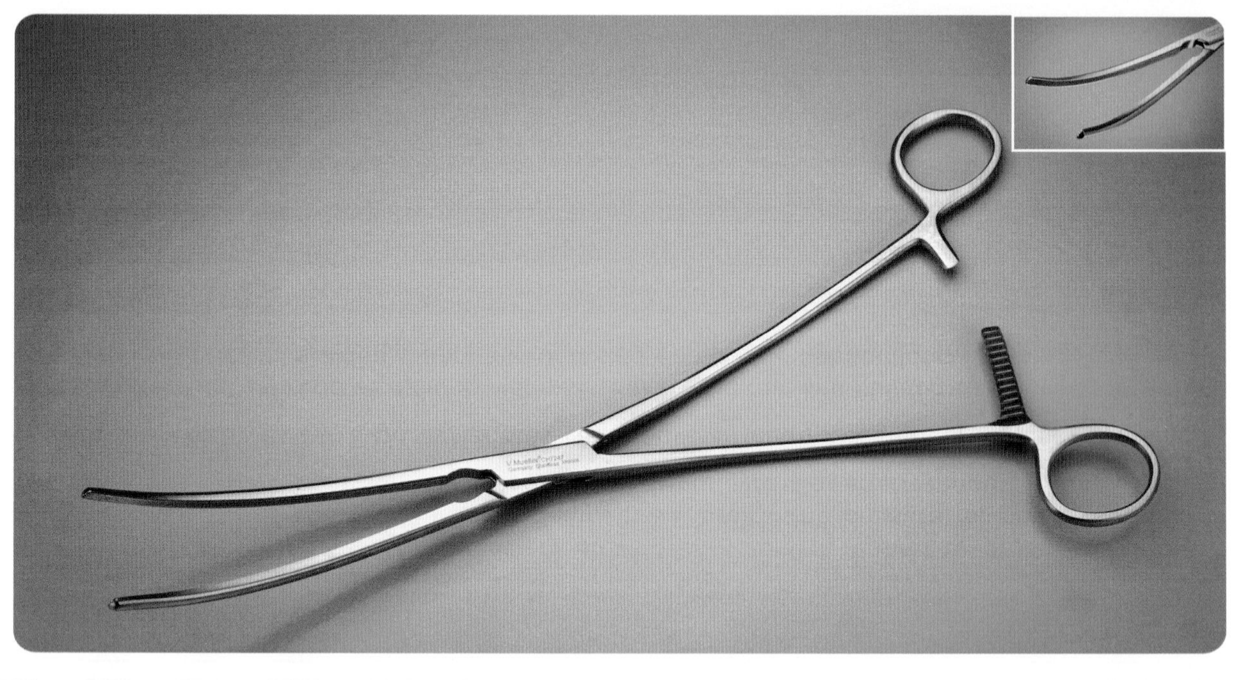

Clamp/Crafoord

USE • To secure hemostasis in cardiovascular and vascular surgery; also used as ligature forceps

VARIETIES • Straight or curved

ALSO KNOWN AS • Coarctation clamp

138

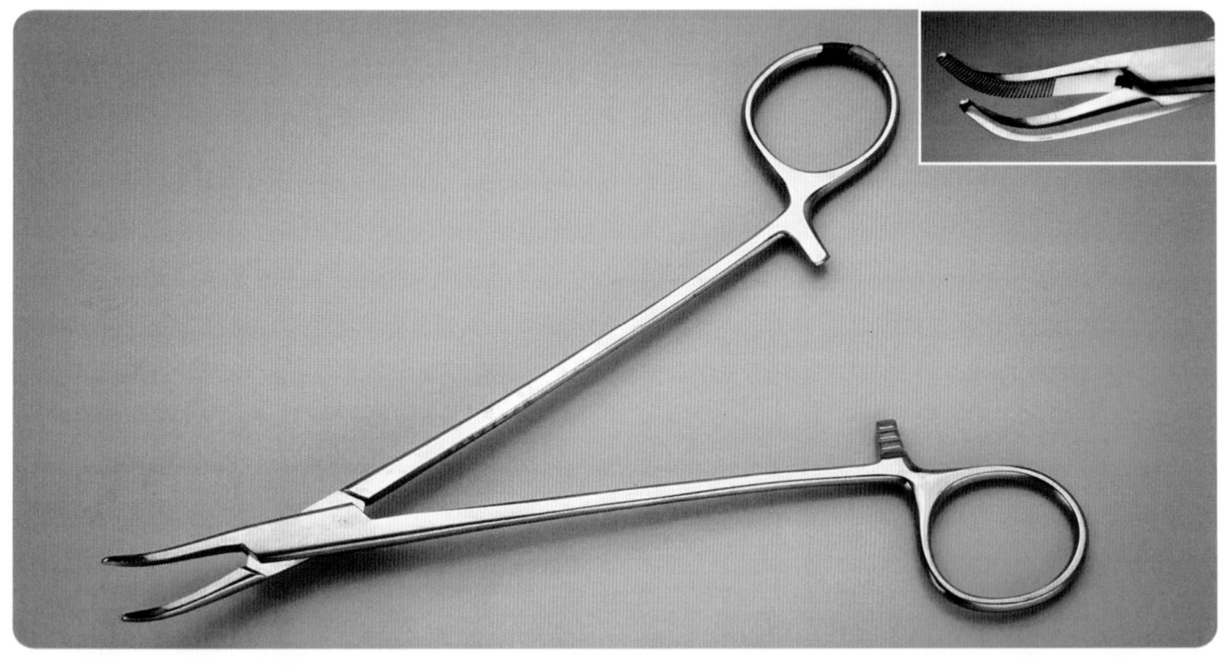

Clamp/Crile

USE • To secure temporary hemostasis in deep anatomy (e.g., for vessel suture)

VARIETIES • Straight or curved; serrated along entire length of jaw; various lengths

ALSO KNOWN AS • Péan clamp, Rankin clamp, Rochester clamp, Schnidt clamp, snap clamp

140

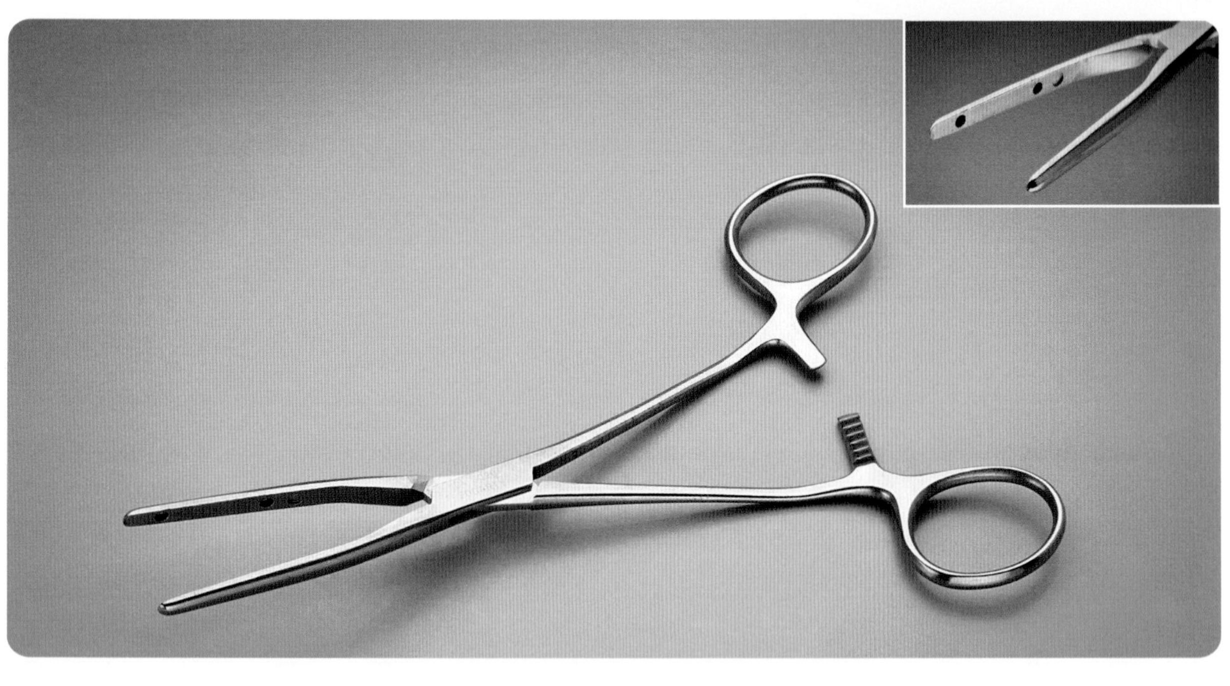

Clamp/Fogarty

USE • To provide complete or partial vessel occlusion

VARIETIES • Noncompressive hydragrip blades; long or short; straight or angled; replaceable soft jaw inserts

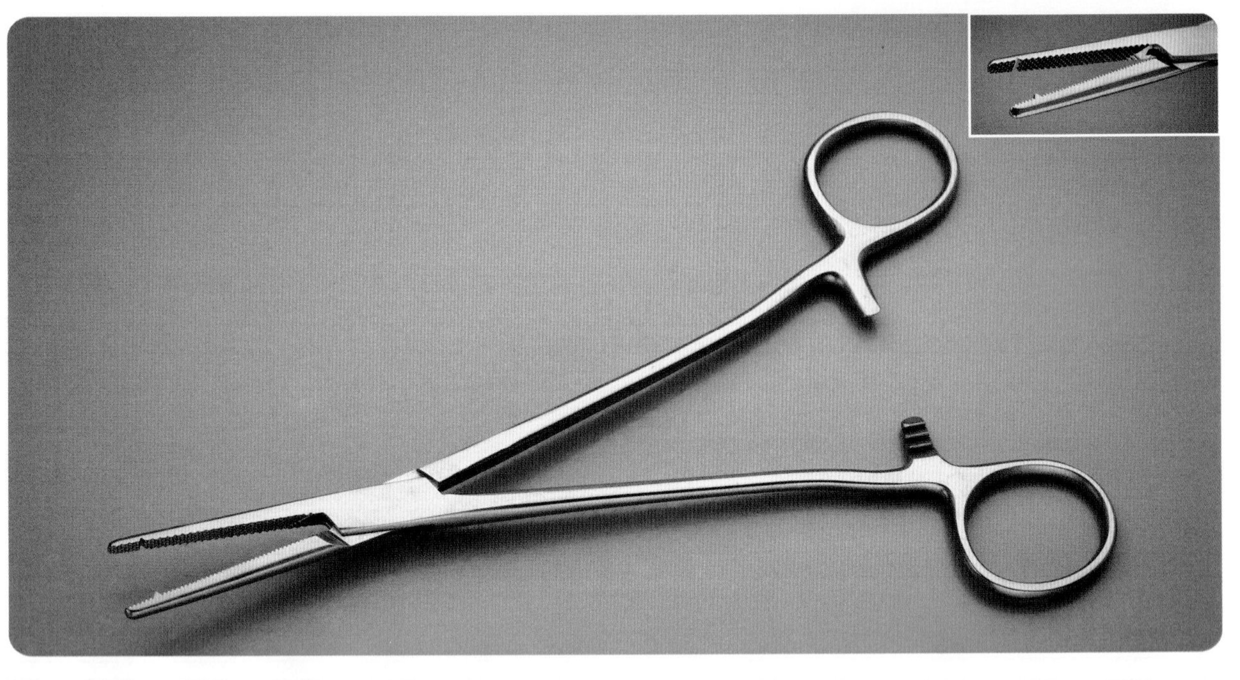

Clamp/Heaney

USE • To provide tissue occlusion during hysterectomy

VARIETIES • Heavy pattern; single tooth; double tooth; longitudinal serrations; curved or straight

ALSO KNOWN AS • Heaney hysterectomy forceps

144

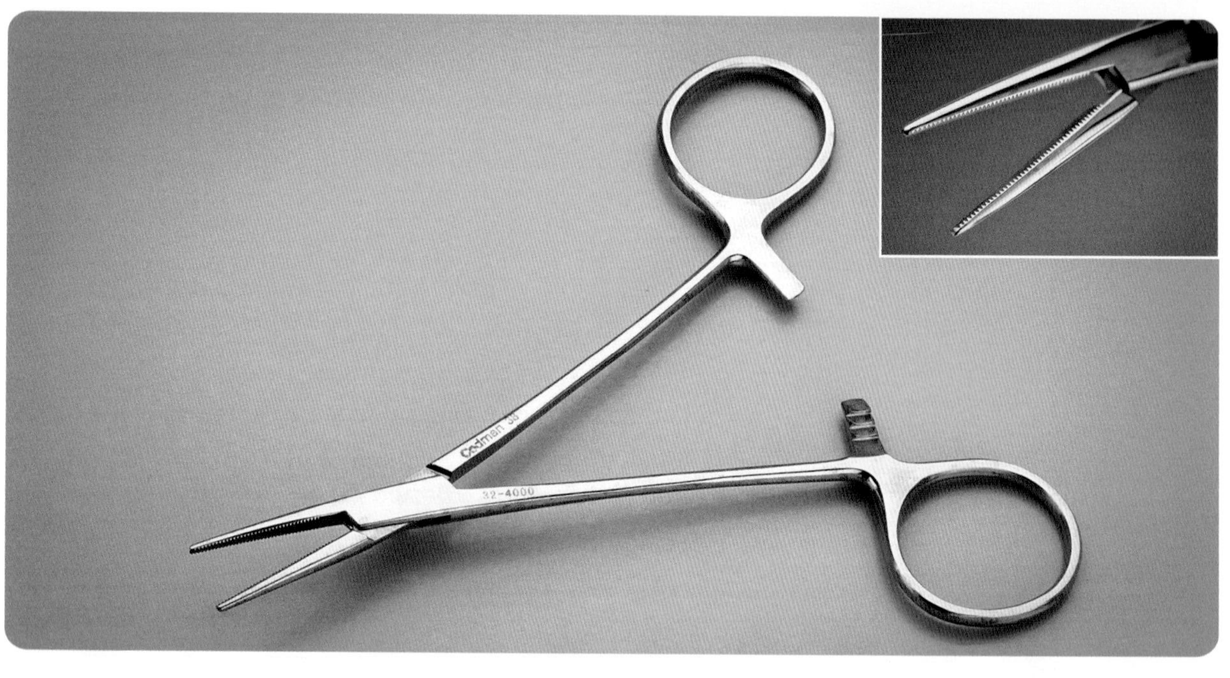

Clamp/Hemostat

USE • To secure individual bleeding vessels for hemostasis

VARIETIES • Straight or curved; serrations along entire length of jaw; about 5½ to 6 inches long

ALSO KNOWN AS • Halsted clamp

146

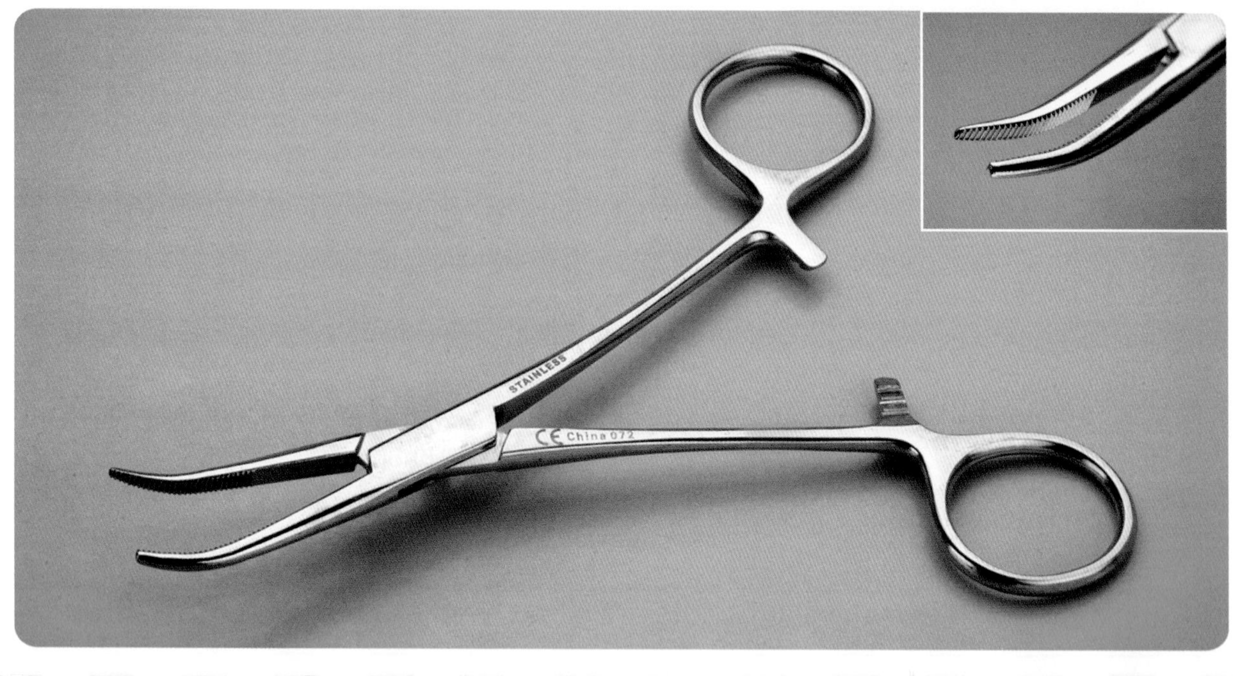

Clamp/Hemostat, Adson

USE • To secure hemostasis of vessels (e.g., in neurosurgery)

VARIETIES • Straight or curved; 7¼ or 8¾ inches long; serrations along half the length of the jaw

148

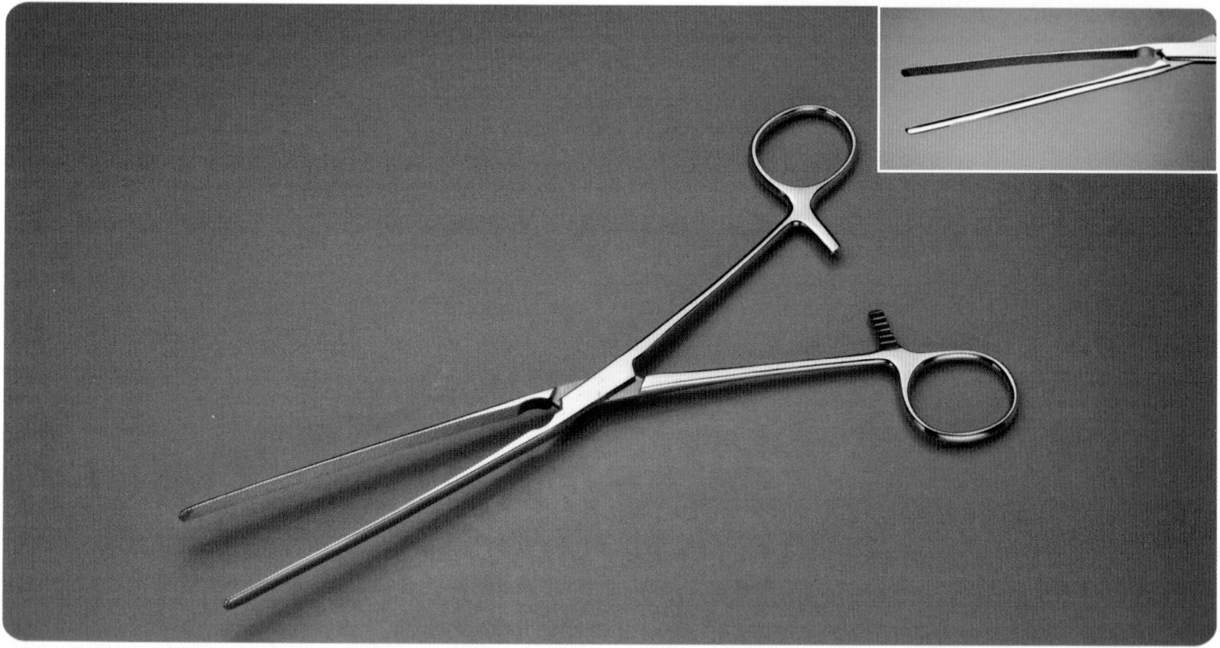

Clamp/Intestinal, Doyen

USE • To control bleeding temporarily during gastrointestinal surgery

VARIETIES • Straight or curved; longitudinal serrations; flexible blades

ALSO KNOWN AS • Doyen intestinal forceps

150

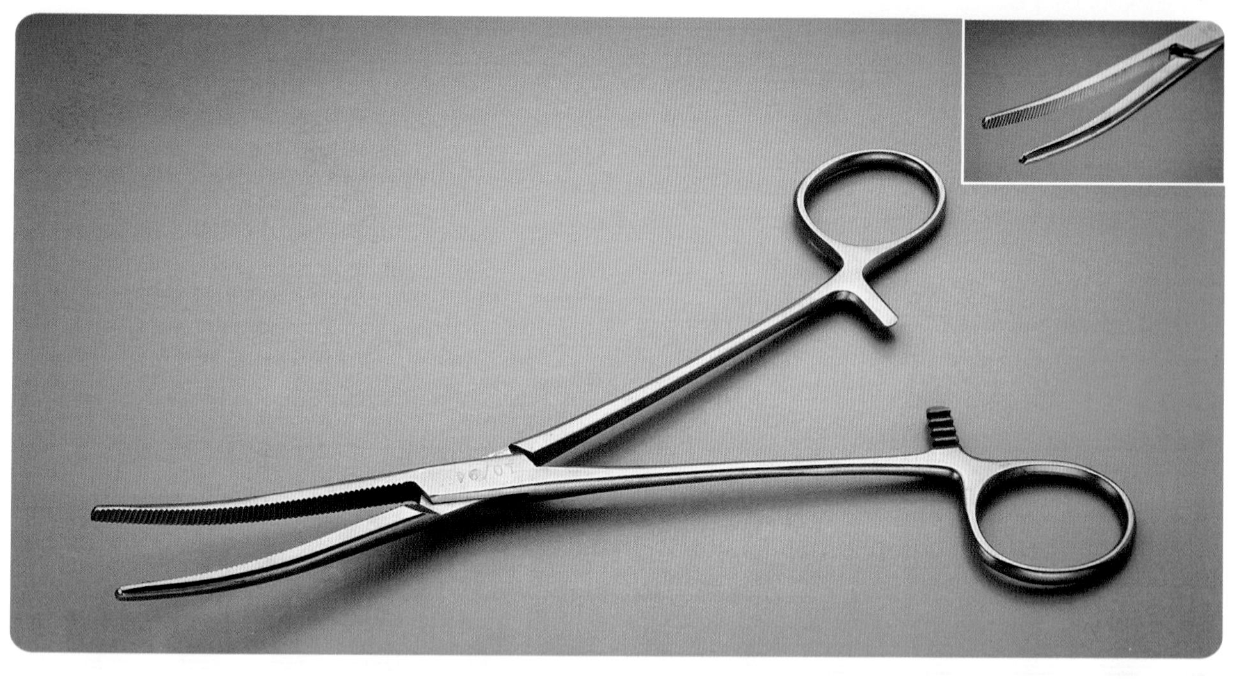

Clamp/Kelly

USE • To clamp bleeding vessels or tissues

VARIETIES • Straight or curved; serrations along part of length of jaw; 5 to 10 inches long

ALSO KNOWN AS • Crile clamp, Péan clamp, Rochester clamp

152

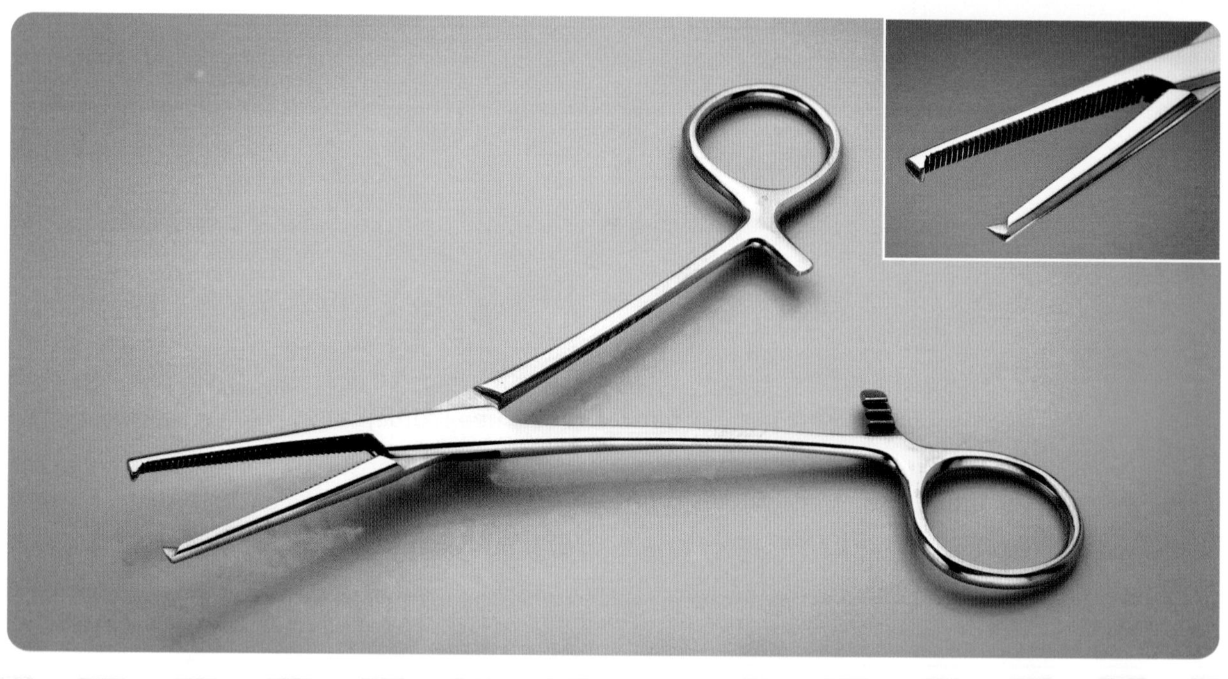

Clamp/Kocher

USE • To secure hemostasis or to grasp tissue (e.g., for fascia approximation)

VARIETIES • Straight or curved; fine or heavy; various lengths

ALSO KNOWN AS • Rochester-Ochsner clamp

154

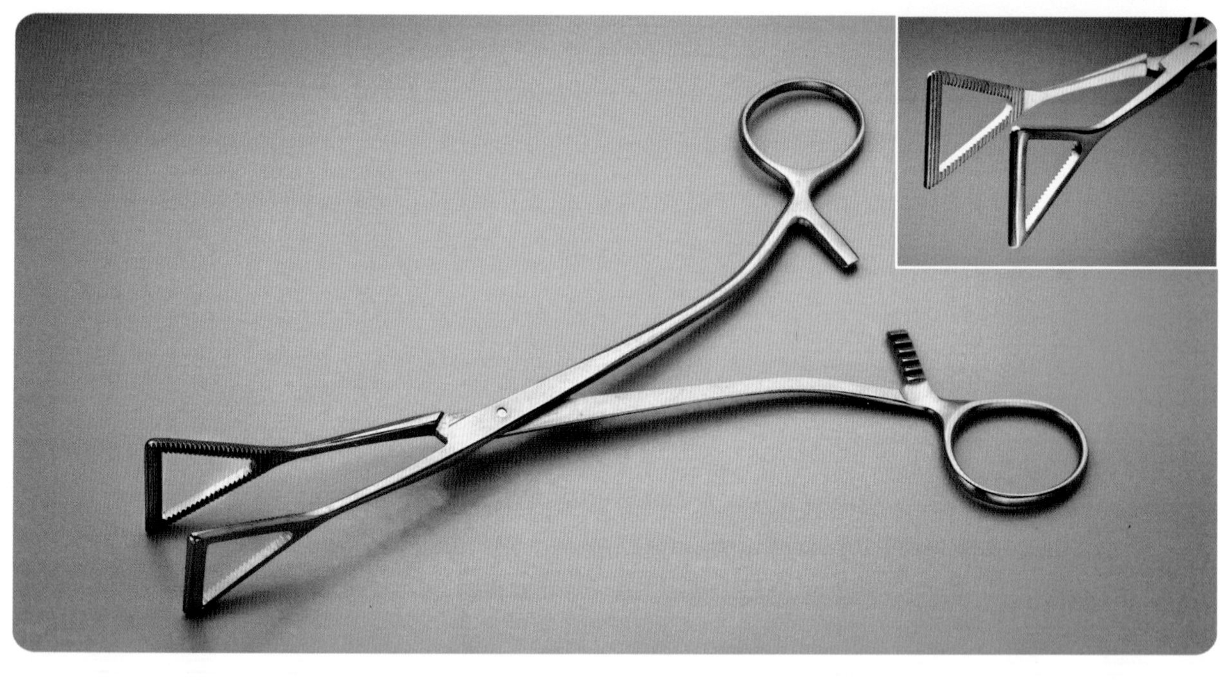

Clamp/Lung, Duval

USE • To hold lung tissue

VARIETIES • Atraumatic; small, medium, or large tip; straight or angled

ALSO KNOWN AS • Collin clamp, Lovelace clamp

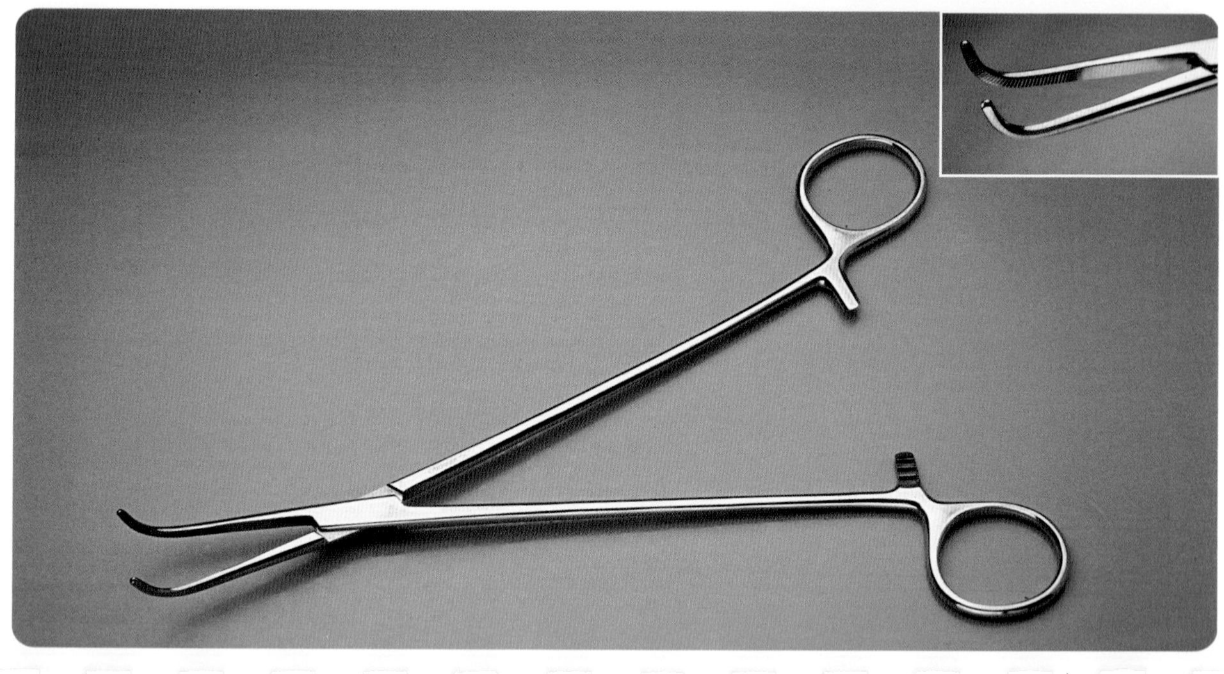

Clamp/Mixter

USE • To secure temporary occlusion of a blood vessel in deep anatomy; to use in general surgery and gynecologic surgery

VARIETIES • Various lengths; a right angle clamp

ALSO KNOWN AS • 90 degree clamp

158

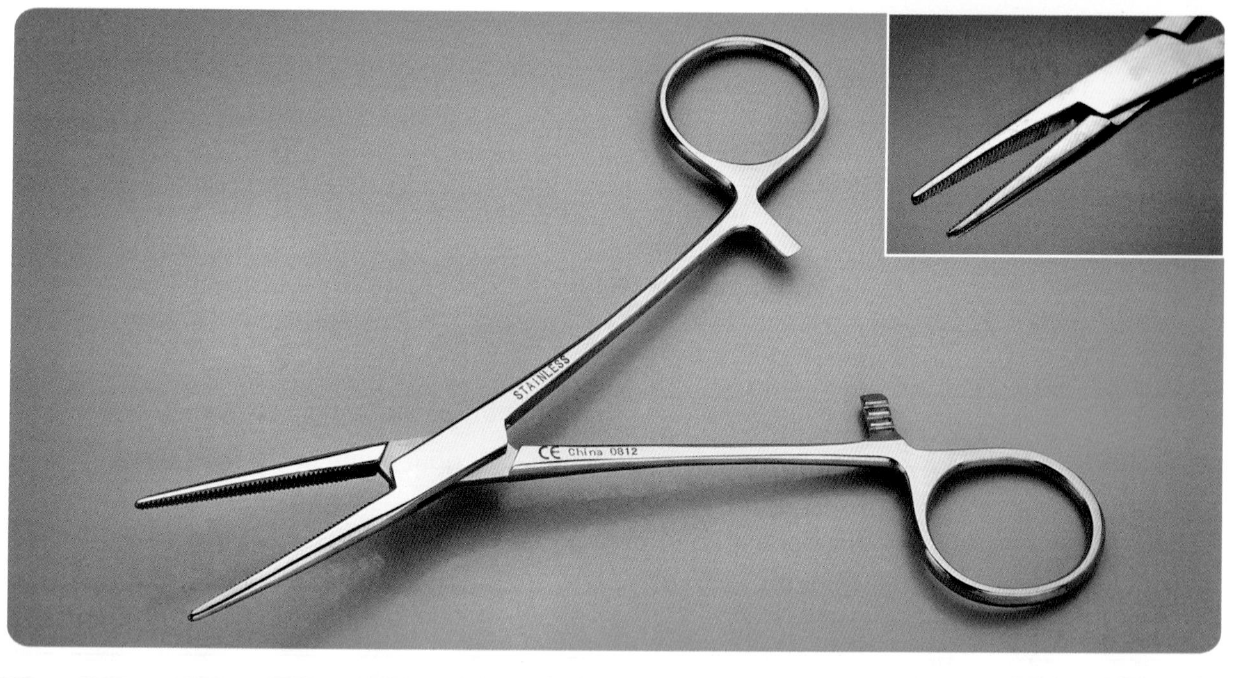

Clamp/Mosquito

USE • To secure hemostasis of delicate tissues (e.g., in plastic surgery and hand surgery)

VARIETIES • Straight or curved; serrations along entire length of jaw; 5 to 5½ inches long

ALSO KNOWN AS • Halsted clamp, snap clamp

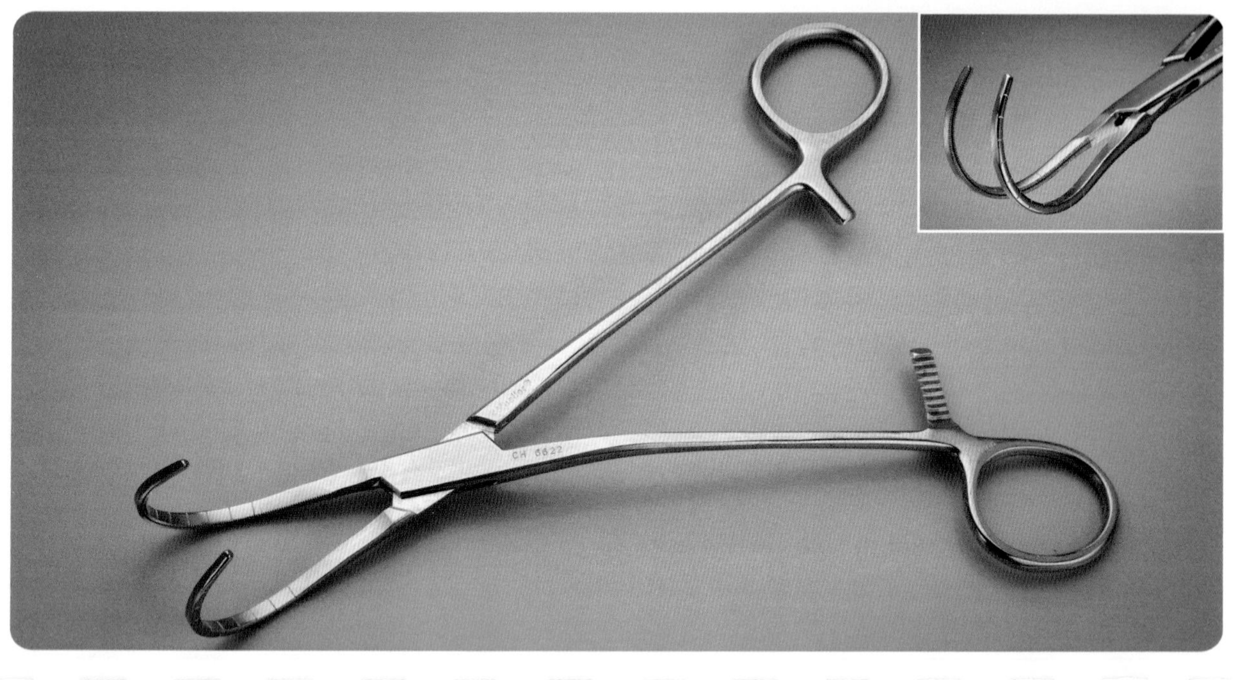
CH 6622

Clamp/Patent Ductus

USE • To secure arterial or venous occlusion during cardiovascular surgery

VARIETIES • Straight; angled slightly or sharply; various lengths

ALSO KNOWN AS • Cooley clamp, Cooley patent ductus clamp, DeBakey clamp, Glover clamp, peripheral vascular clamp, vena cava clamp

162

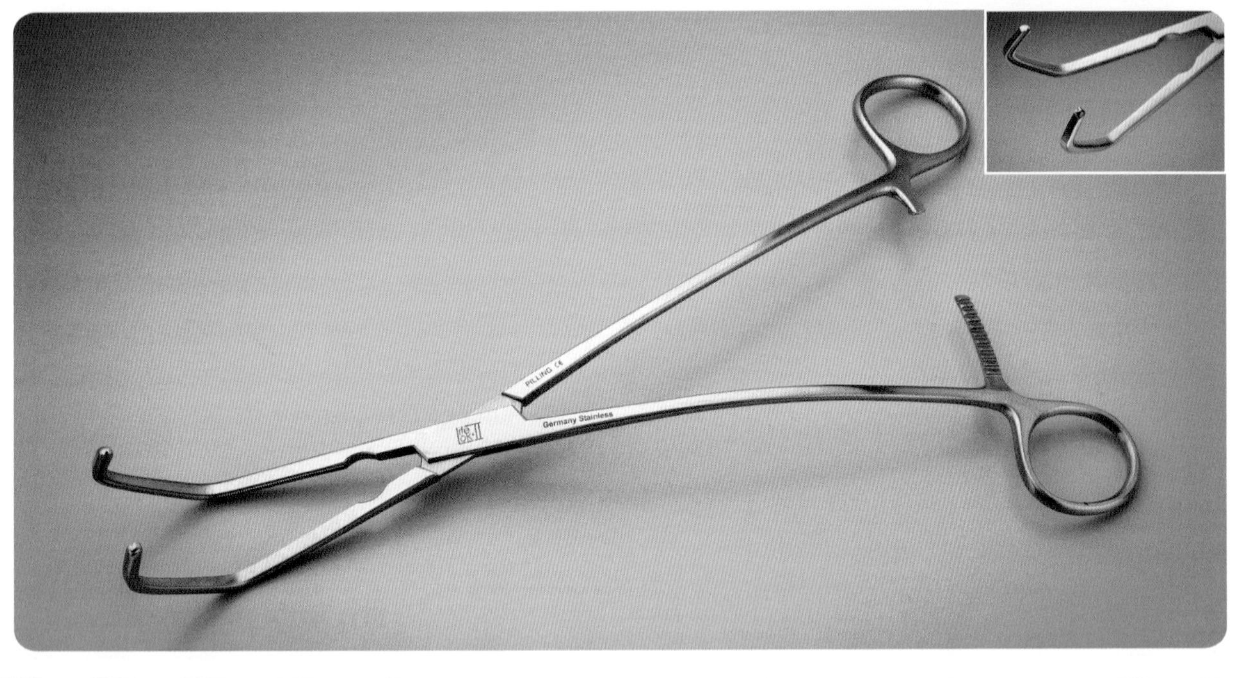

Clamp/Satinsky

USE • To secure partial vessel occlusion during cardiovascular and vascular surgery

VARIETIES • Small, medium, or large angled jaws; about 10 inches long overall

ALSO KNOWN AS • Aortic clamp, DeBakey-Satinsky vena cava clamp, side-biting clamp

164

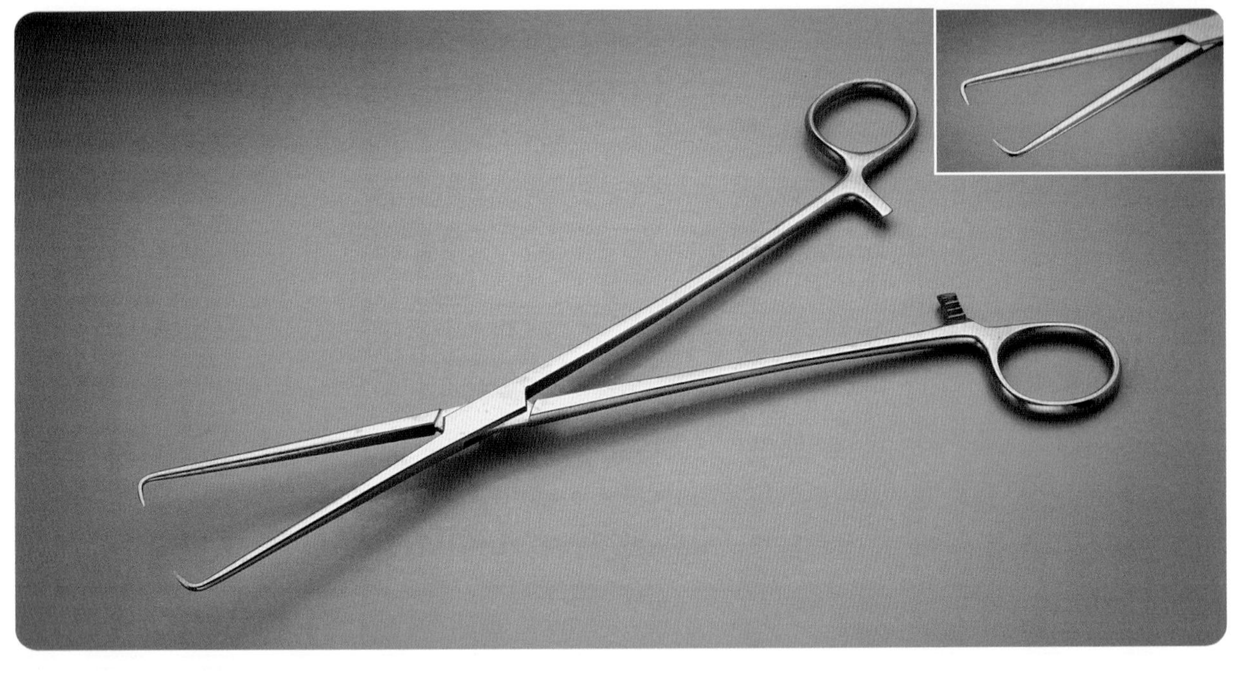

Clamp/Tenaculum, Uterine

USE • To grasp the cervix and apply traction to the uterus

VARIETIES • Straight or curved; single, double, or triple tooth; 5½ to 10 inches long

ALSO KNOWN AS • Adair clamp, Barrett clamp, Braun clamp, Duplay clamp, Jarcho clamp, Kahn clamp, Schroeder clamp, Stauder clamp

166

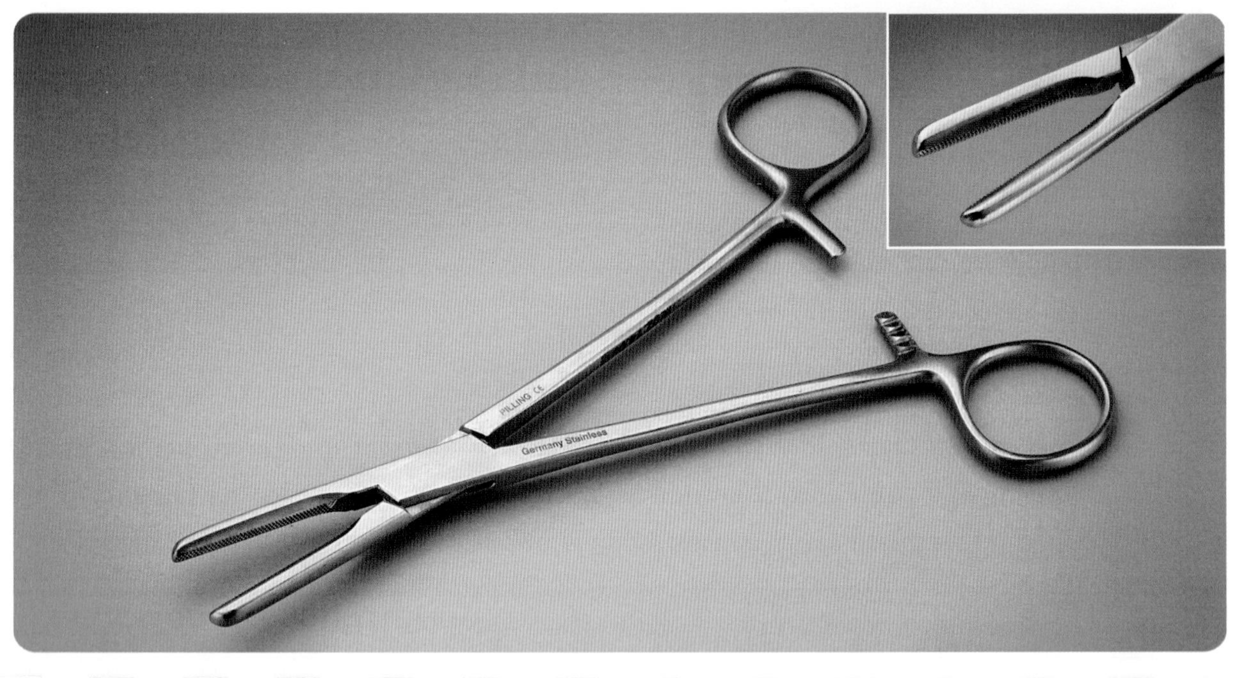

Clamp/Tubing

USE • To occlude a tube (e.g., during extracorporeal circulation)

VARIETIES • Straight, serrated jaws with or without guard; sized to fit various tubing diameters; 6½ to 8 inches long

ALSO KNOWN AS • Tube occluding clamp

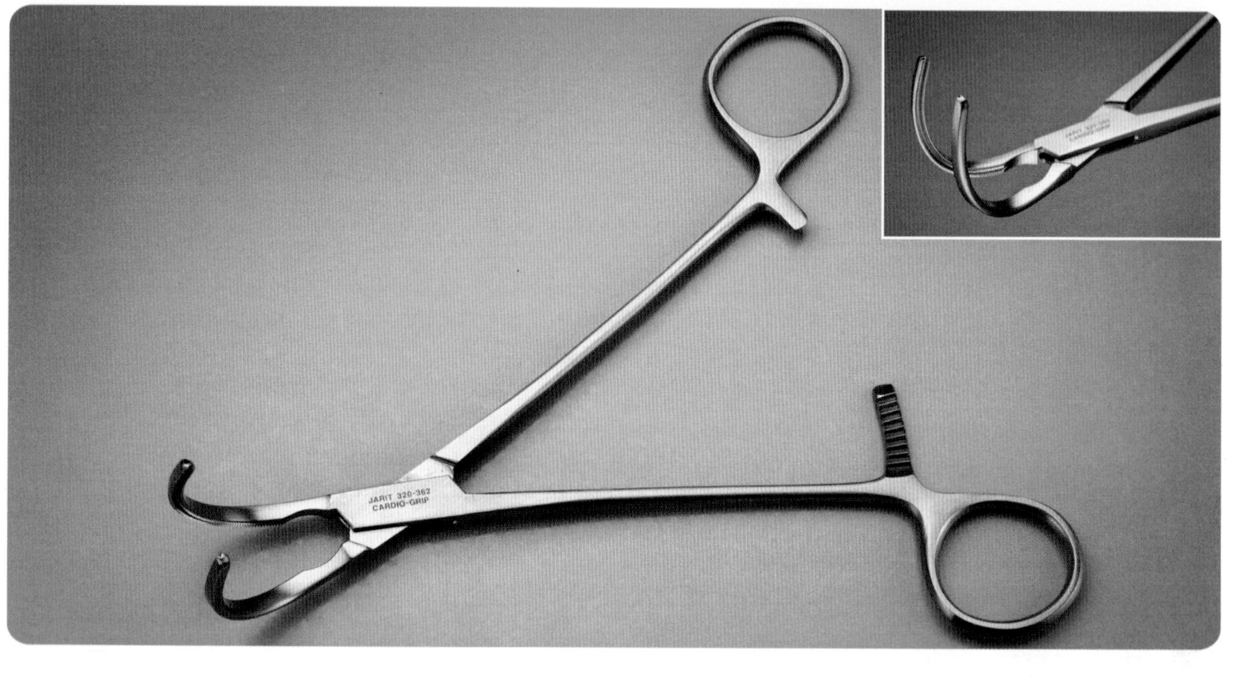
JARIT 320-362
CARDIO-GRIP

Clamp/Vascular, Glover

USE • To secure hemostasis during cardiovascular surgery

VARIETIES • Straight or angular; 3 or 6 cm jaws; various lengths

ALSO KNOWN AS • Glover coarctation clamp, Glover patent ductus clamp

170

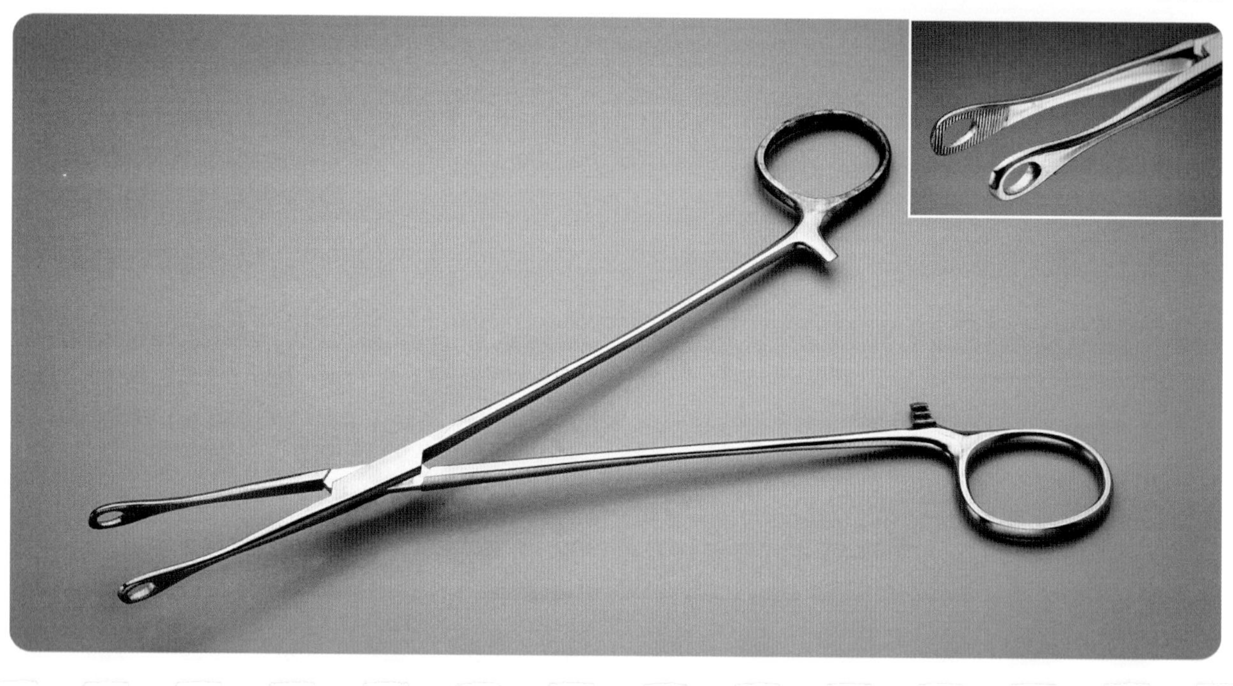

Clamp/Williams

USE • To secure tissue or organs during gynecologic infertility surgery on fallopian tubes and ovaries

VARIETIES • Fenestrated jaws with cross-serrated tips; about 6½ inches long

ALSO KNOWN AS • Williams uterine forceps

172

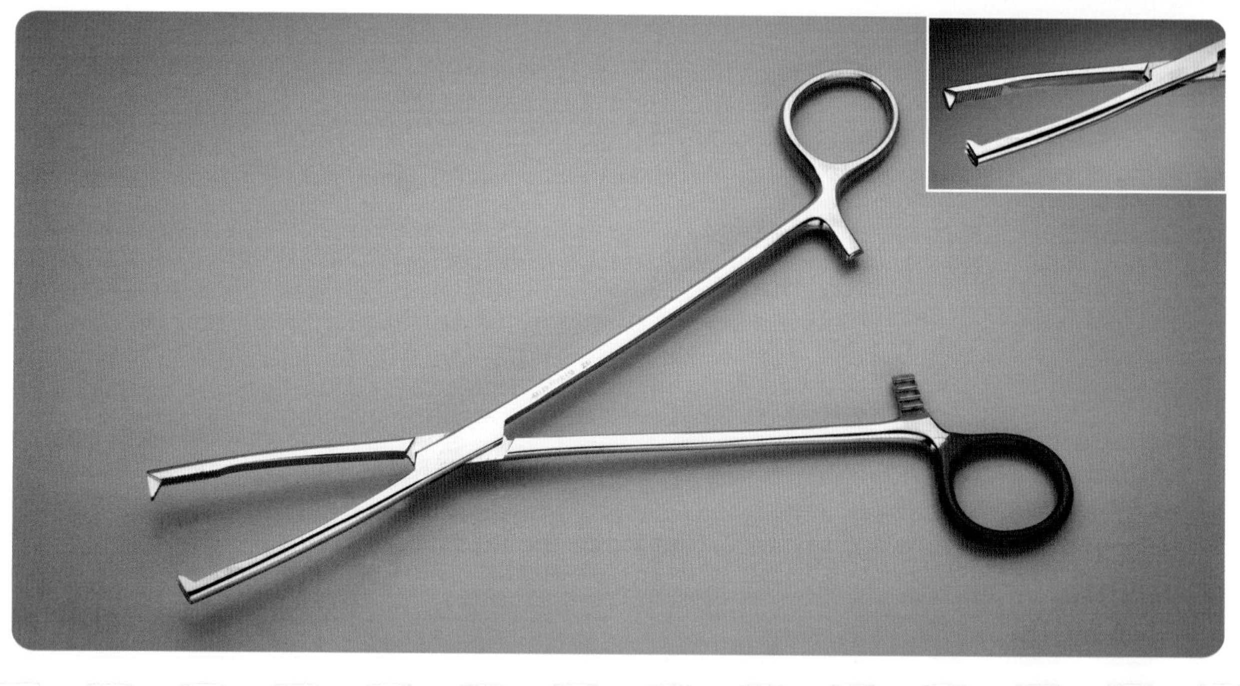

Tenaculum/Uterine, Jacob

USE • To grasp uterus

VARIETIES • Traumatic; straight or curved; serrated jaws; 2 × 2 teeth; 8½ inches long

ALSO KNOWN AS • Jacob tenaculum, Schroeder vulsellum forceps

CHAPTER 4 Retractors

Retractors are surgical instruments that separate the edges of a surgical incision or wound and hold back underlying organs and tissues so that body parts under an incision can be accessed. Retractors assist in visualizing the operative field while preventing trauma to other tissue. They are also used to spread open skin, ribs, and other tissues.

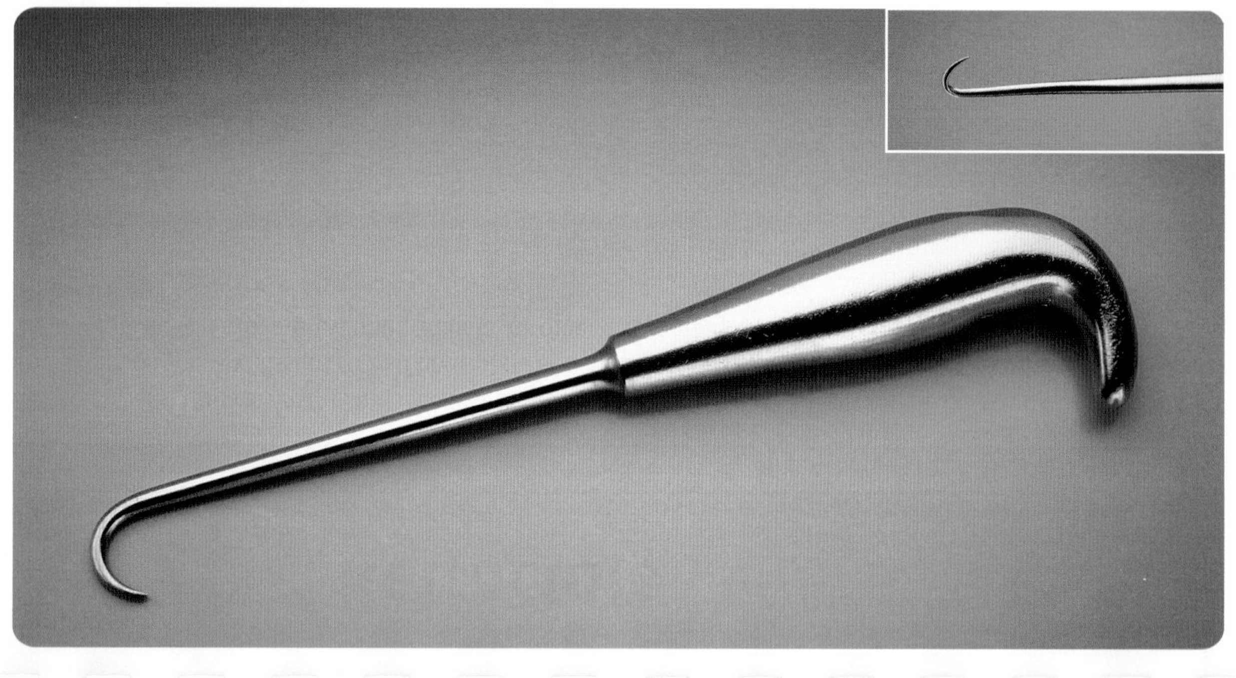

Hook/Bone

USE • To grasp bone in order to apply traction during orthopedic surgery

VARIETIES • Sharp or blunt; 7 or 9 inches long

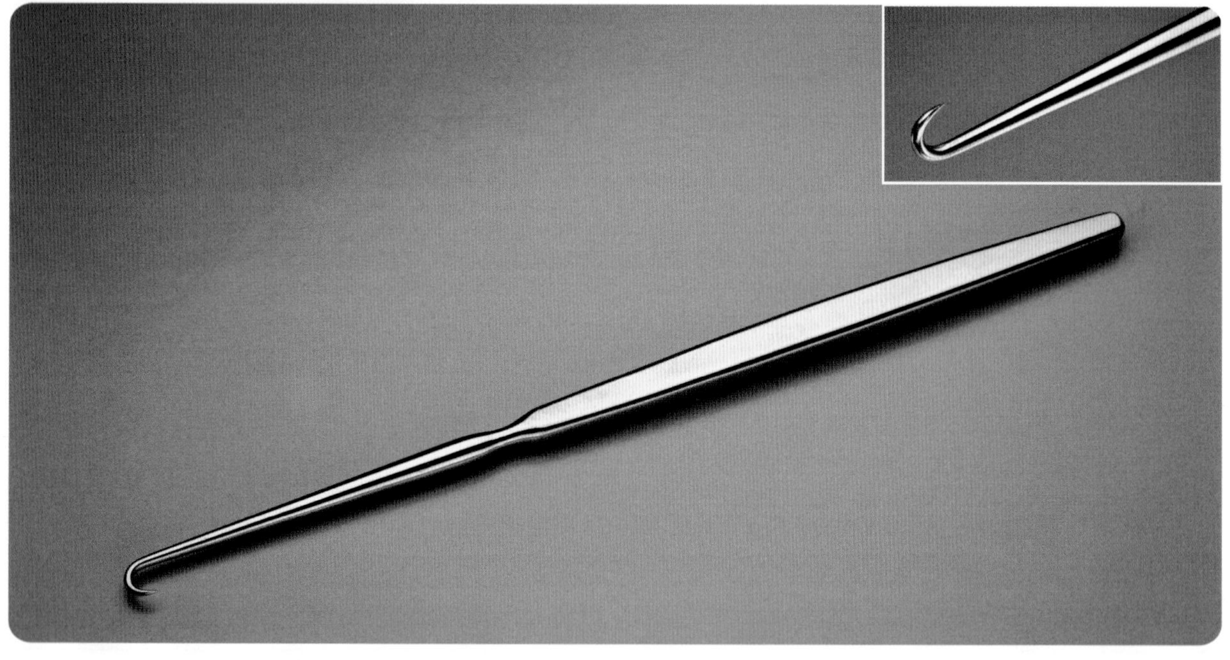

Hook/Dural

USE • To hold dura mater during neurosurgery

VARIETIES • Sharp or blunt; various lengths

ALSO KNOWN AS • Adson dural hook (8 inches), Frazier dural hook (6 inches)

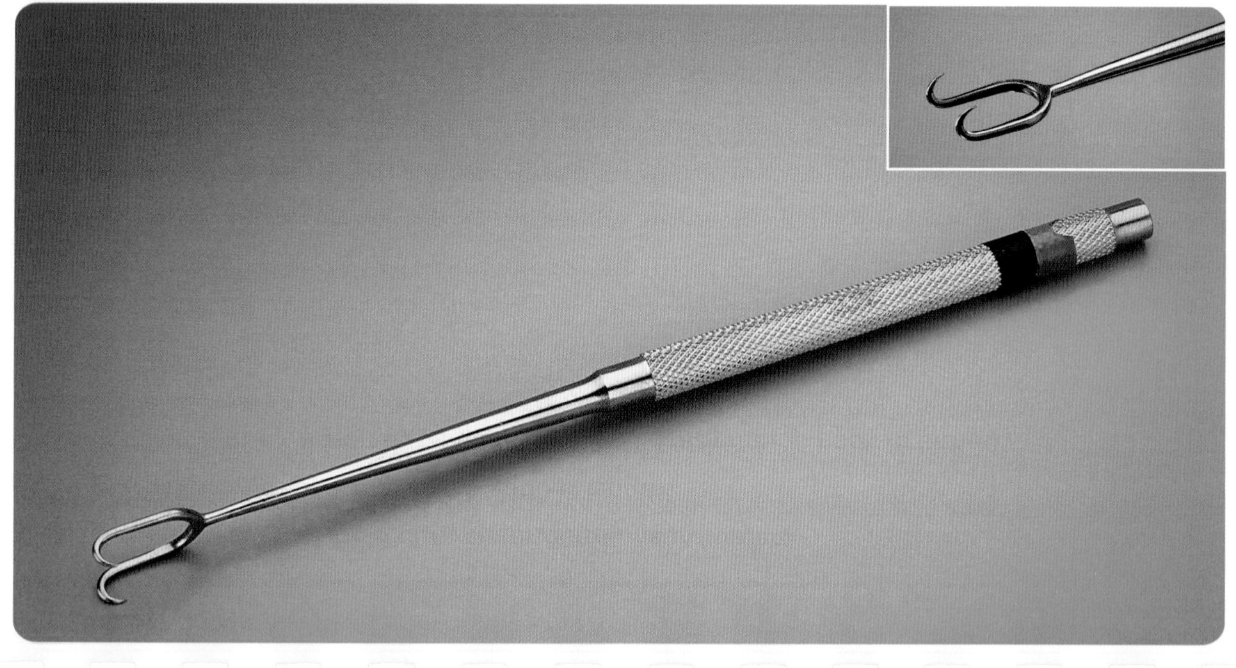

Hook/Guthrie

USE • To retract skin during plastic surgery

VARIETIES • Various lengths; sharp or blunt prongs

ALSO KNOWN AS • Cottle double hook, Joseph hook, skin hook

182

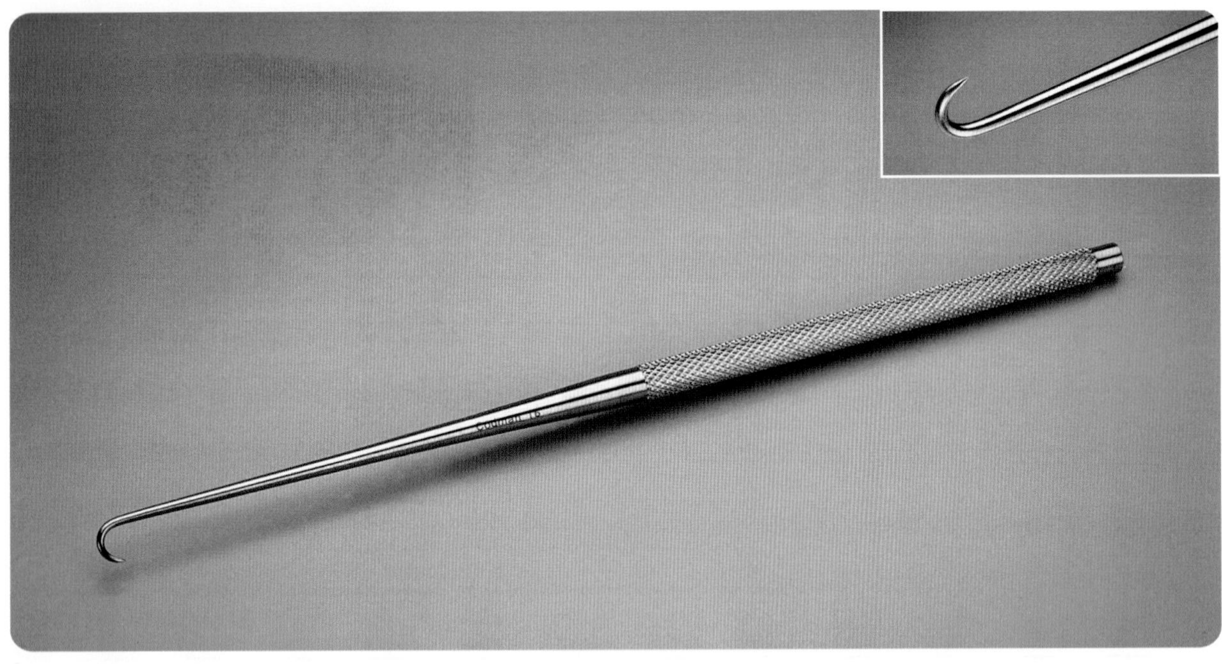

Hook/Skin

USE • To retract dermis during plastic surgery

VARIETIES • Single or double hook; sharp or blunt; 5⅜ to 7½ inches long

ALSO KNOWN AS • Cottle skin hook, Freer skin hook, Gillies skin hook, Kleinert-Kutz hook, single hook

184

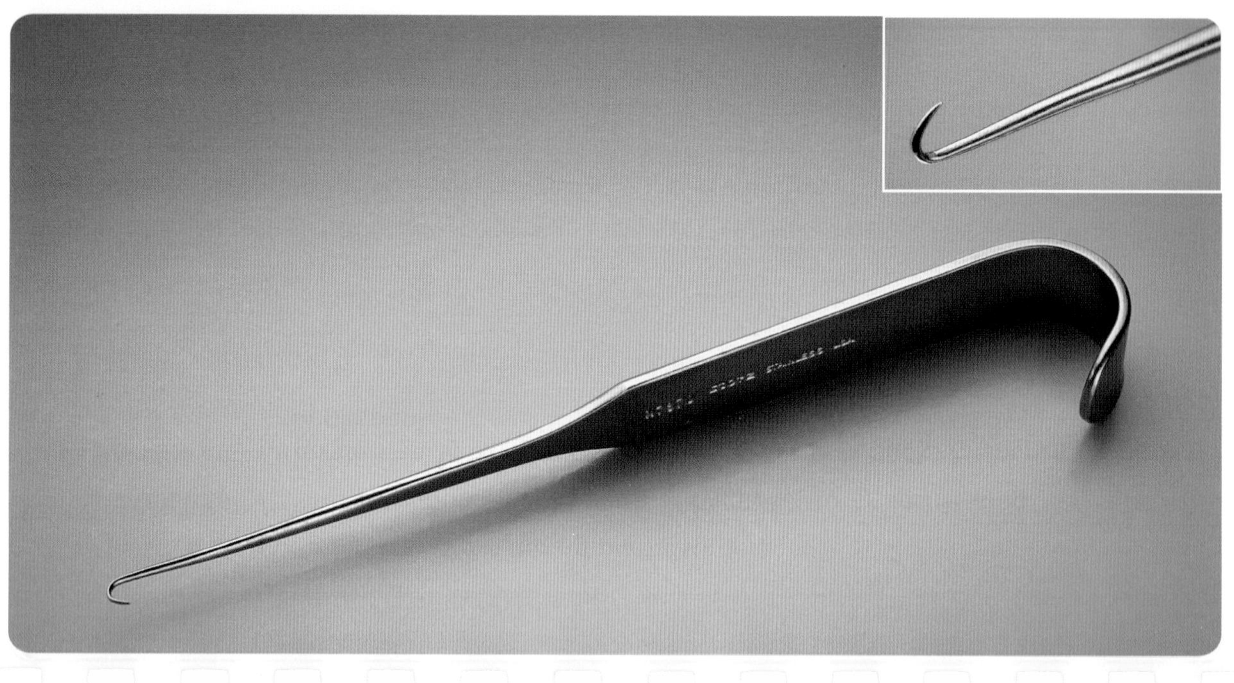

Hook/Tracheal

USE • To grasp and apply traction to tracheal cartilage during tracheostomy; to use with tracheal dilator

VARIETIES • 5 to 6½ inches long; sharp point

ALSO KNOWN AS • Jackson tracheal hook, new tracheal hook

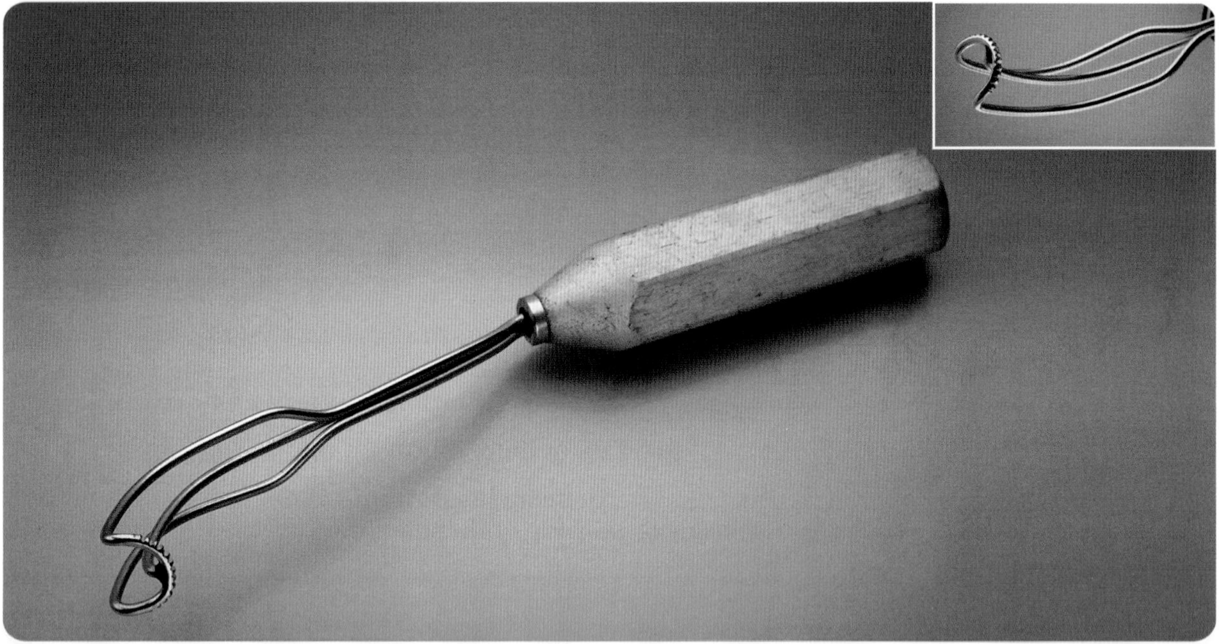

186

Retractor/Aortic Valve

USE • To maintain traction and exposure during open heart surgery; valve replacement procedures

VARIETIES • Various blade widths and depths

ALSO KNOWN AS • Cooley retractor, mitral valve retractor

188

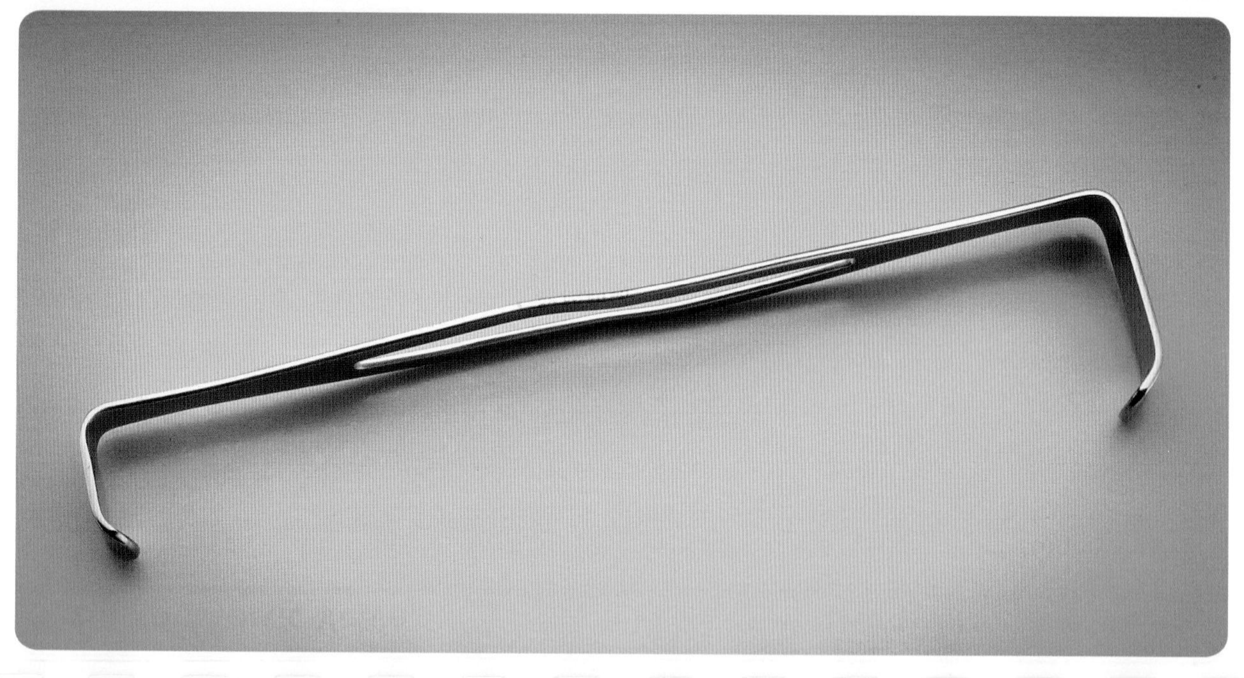

Retractor/Army-Navy

USE	• To maintain wound exposure (handheld)
VARIETIES	• One size (8 inches); usually in pairs
ALSO KNOWN AS	• US Army retractor, USA retractor

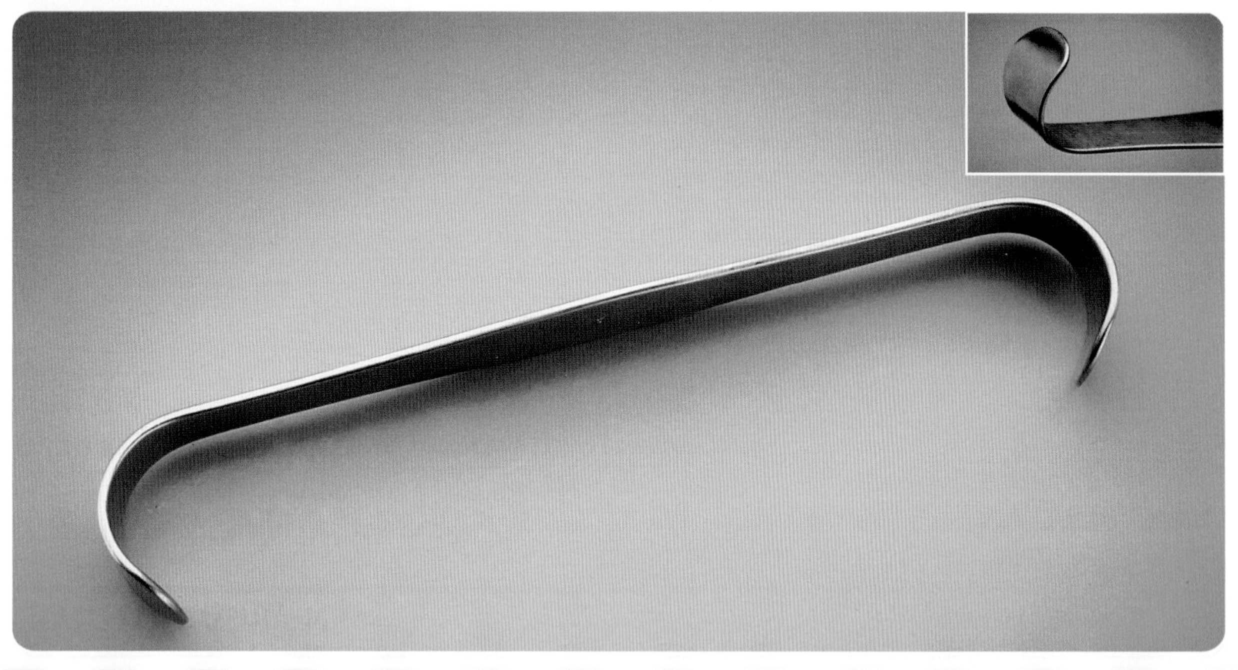

Retractor/Band

USE • To retract soft tissue for wound exposure (handheld)

VARIETIES • Set of two lengths, 5 inches and 7¼ inches; set of two, double-ended

ALSO KNOWN AS • Parker retractor, Parker-Bard retractor

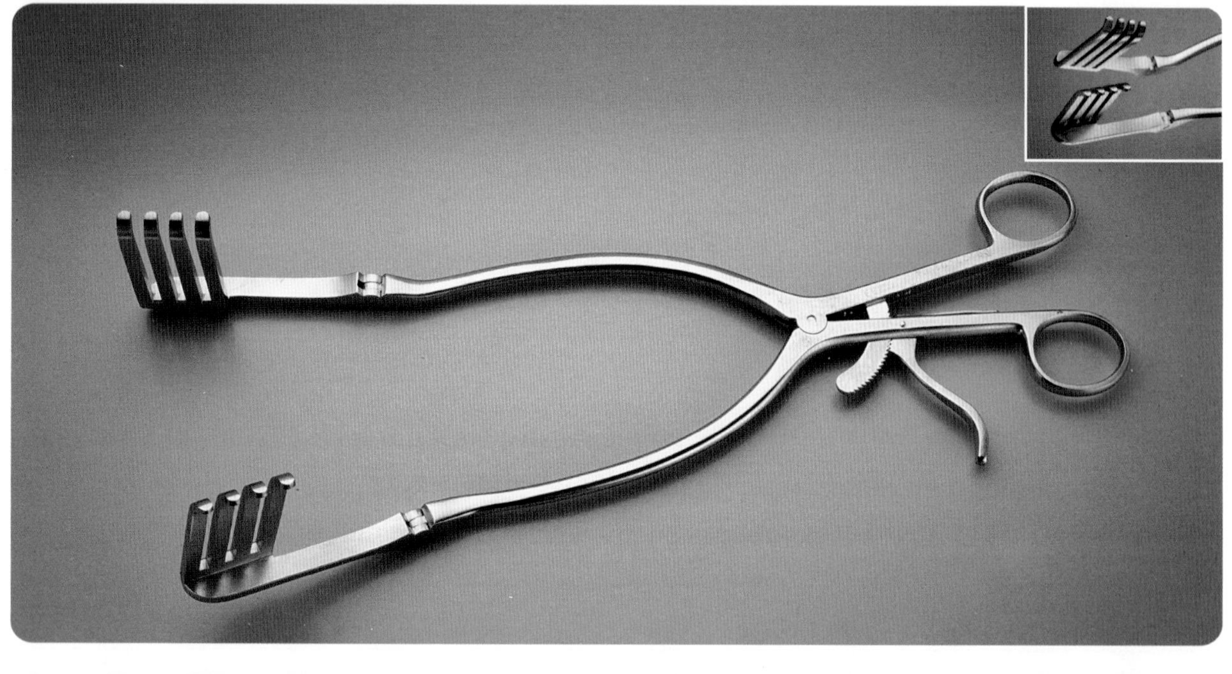

Retractor/Beckman

USE • To maintain wound exposure (self-retaining)

VARIETIES • Sharp or blunt prongs; 4 × 4 or 3 × 4 prongs; various lengths; hinged arms

ALSO KNOWN AS • Beckman goiter retractor, Beckman-Adson retractor, Weitlaner retractor

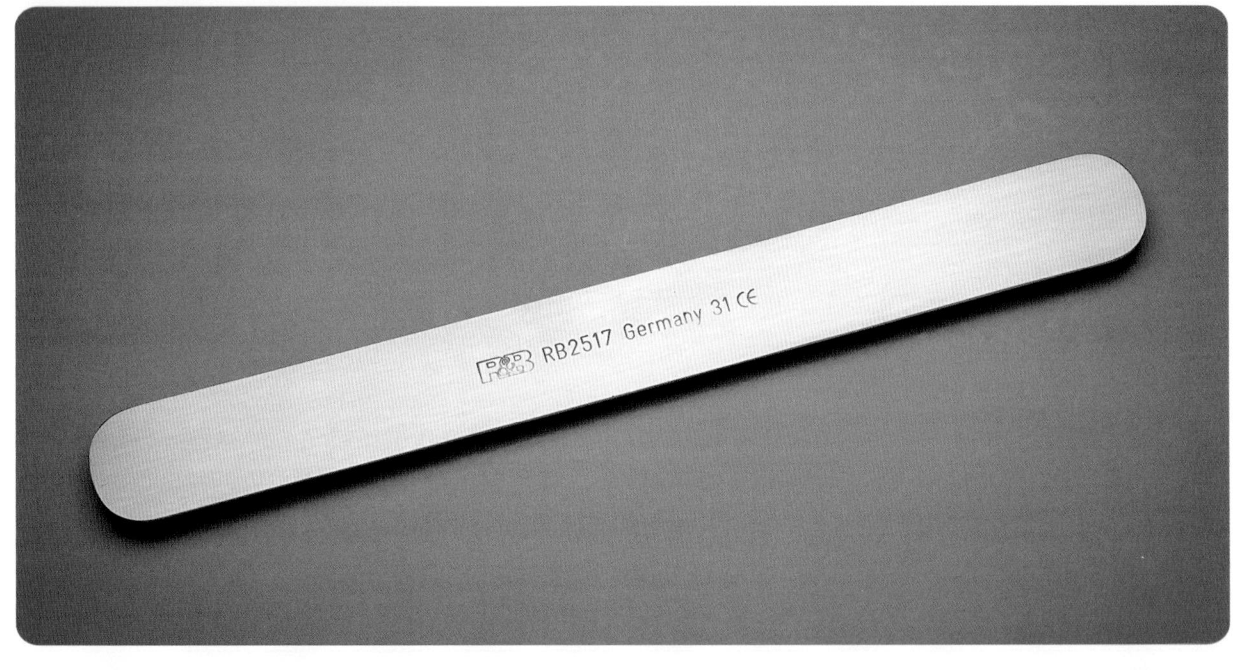
R&B RB2517 Germany 31 CE

Retractor/Brain

USE • To retract brain tissue during craniotomy

VARIETIES • Malleable or S-shaped; various lengths and widths; sometimes coated with silicone to avoid sticking to tissue

ALSO KNOWN AS • Cherry retractor, Cushing retractor, Davis retractor, French retractor, ribbon retractor

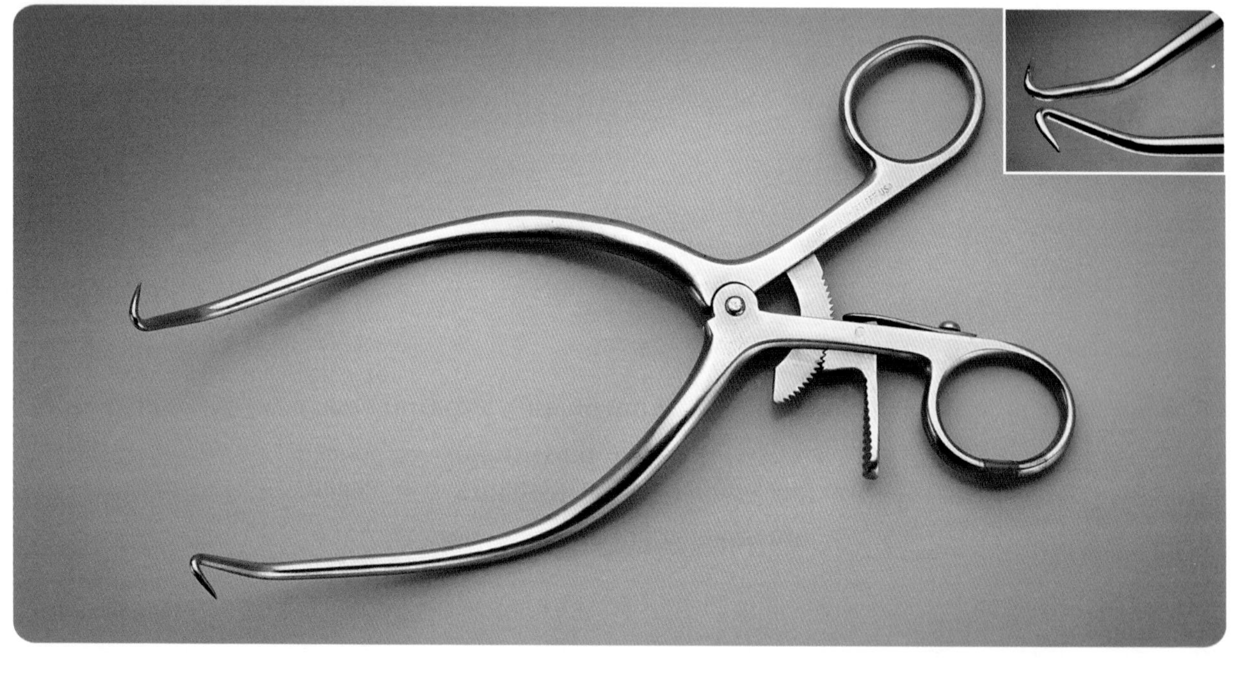

Retractor/Gelpi

USE • To maintain wound exposure during neurosurgery (self-retaining), orthopedic surgery, and neck surgery

VARIETIES • Various lengths; with or without grip lock

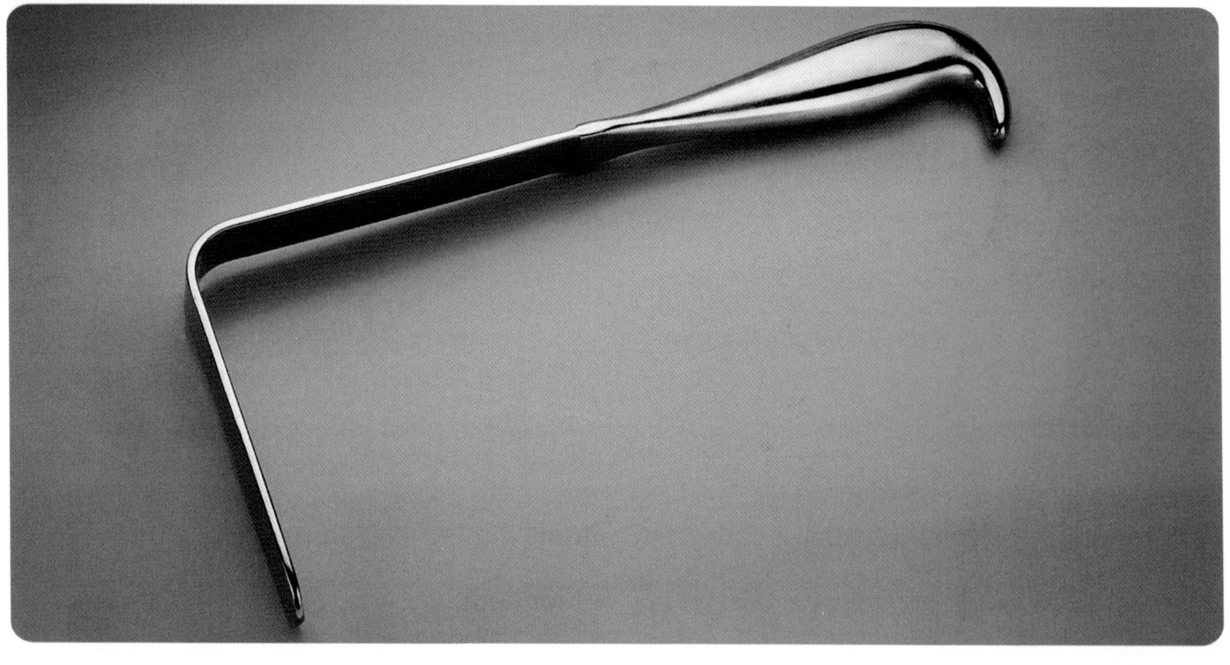

Retractor/Heaney

USE • To retract uterine ligaments for wound exposure during hysterectomy

VARIETIES • Small, medium, or large blades

ALSO KNOWN AS • Right-angled retractor

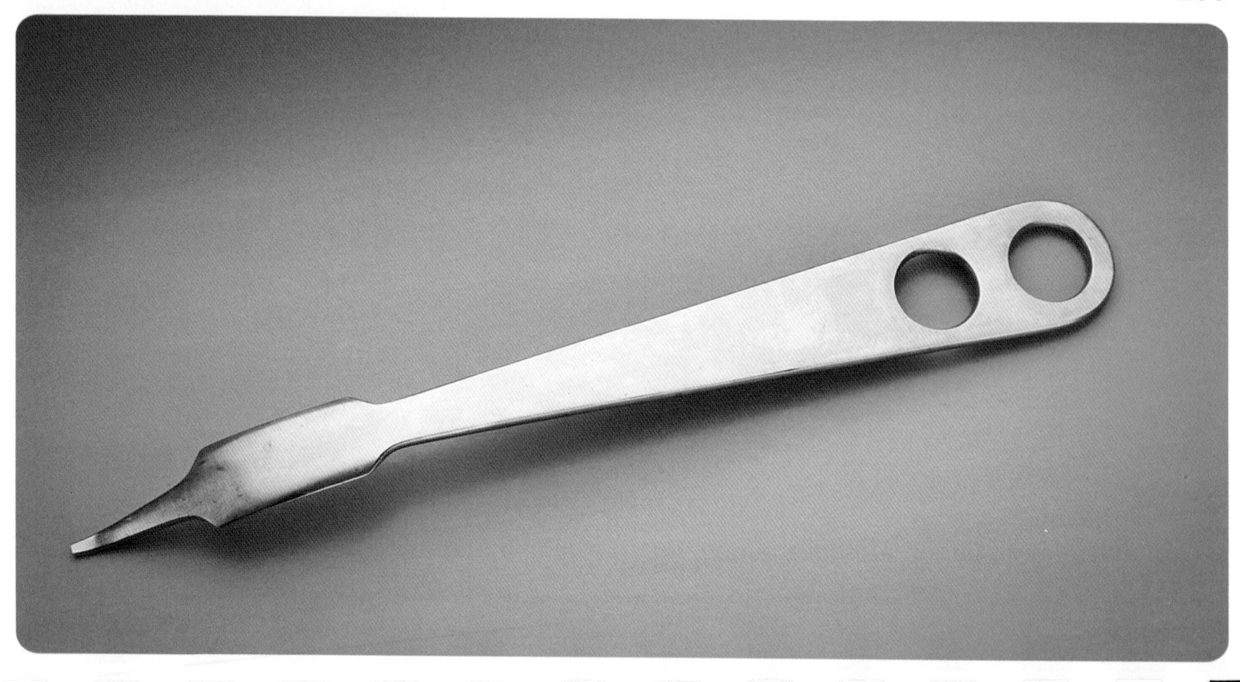

Retractor/Hohmann

USE • To maintain exposure of bone during hip surgery (handheld)

VARIETIES • Blades 6 to 7 mm wide; 6¼ or 9¾ inches long

ALSO KNOWN AS • Cobra retractor

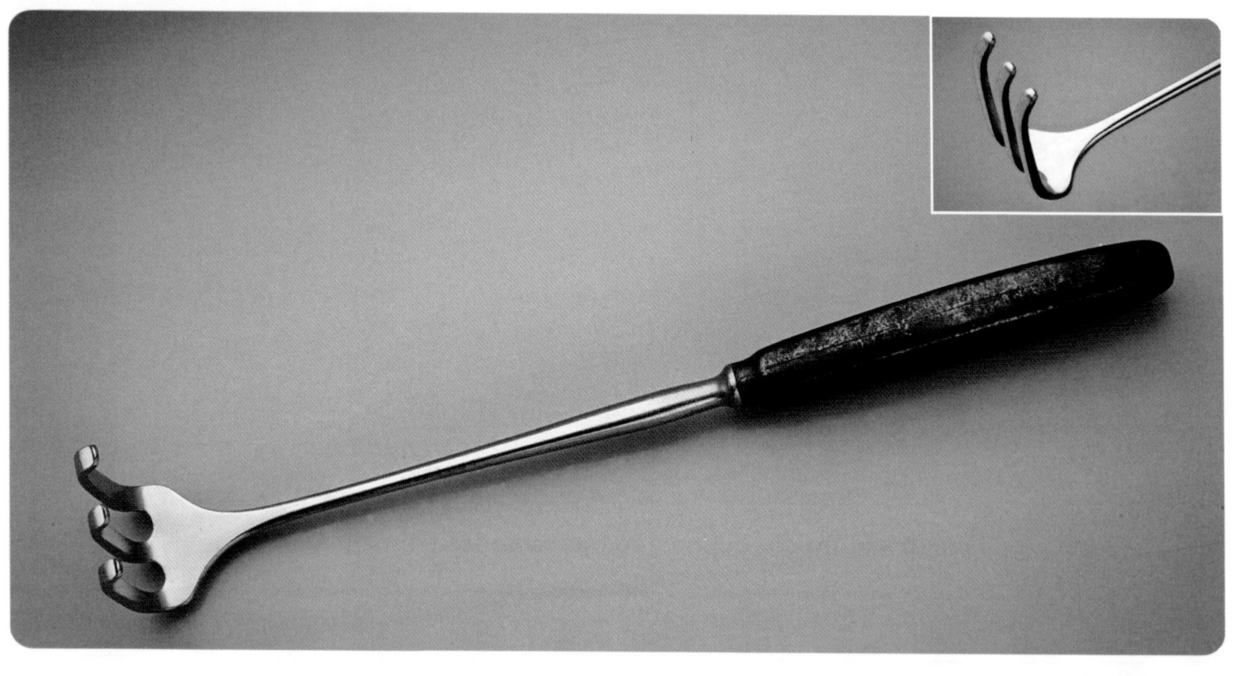

Retractor/Israel

USE • To maintain exposure during hip surgery (handheld)

VARIETIES • Blunt; three to five prongs

ALSO KNOWN AS • Israel rake, large rake

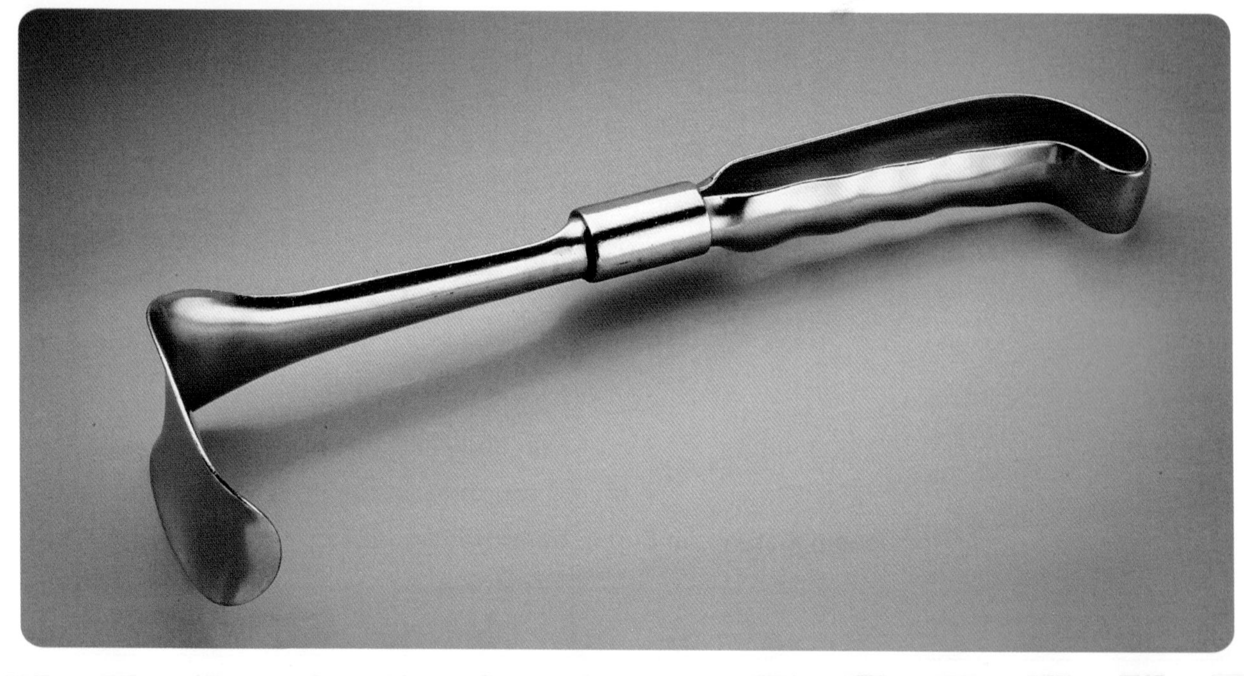

Retractor/Kelly

USE • To maintain wound exposure

VARIETIES • Small (38 × 50 mm), medium (50 × 62 mm), large (62 × 76 mm), or extra large (76 × 88 mm) blades

ALSO KNOWN AS • Single-ended Richardson

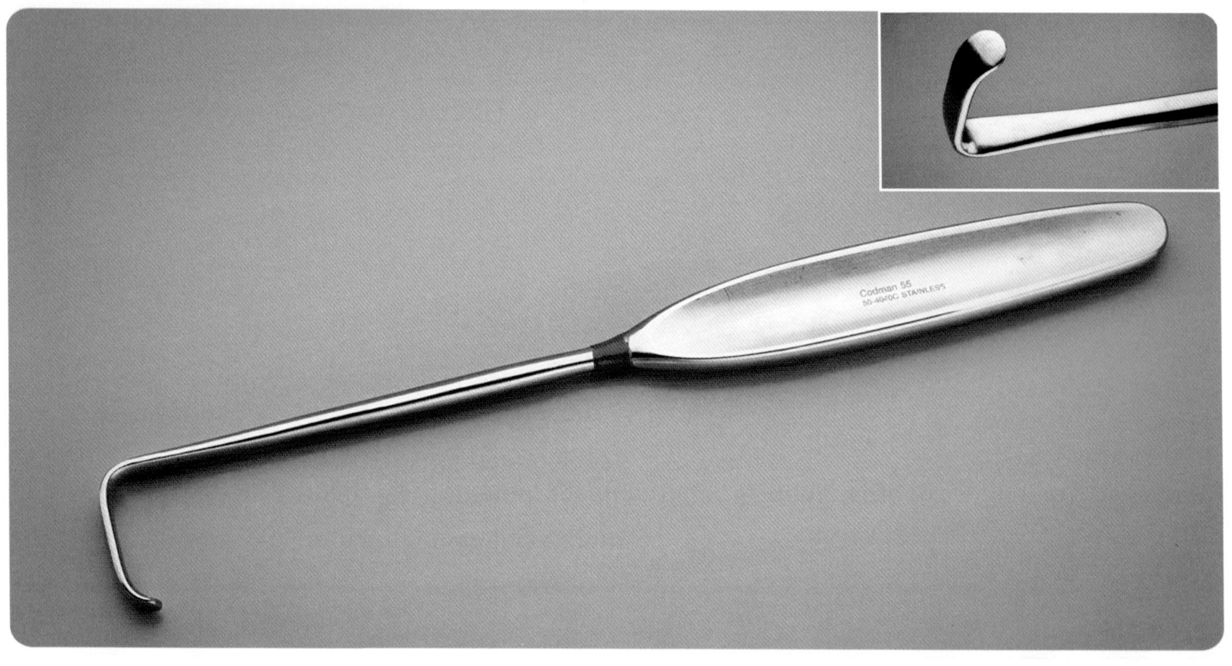
Codman 55
50-4040C STAINLESS

Retractor/Langenbeck

USE • To maintain exposure during plastic surgery or general surgery as a handheld right-angle retractor

VARIETIES • Various blade sizes

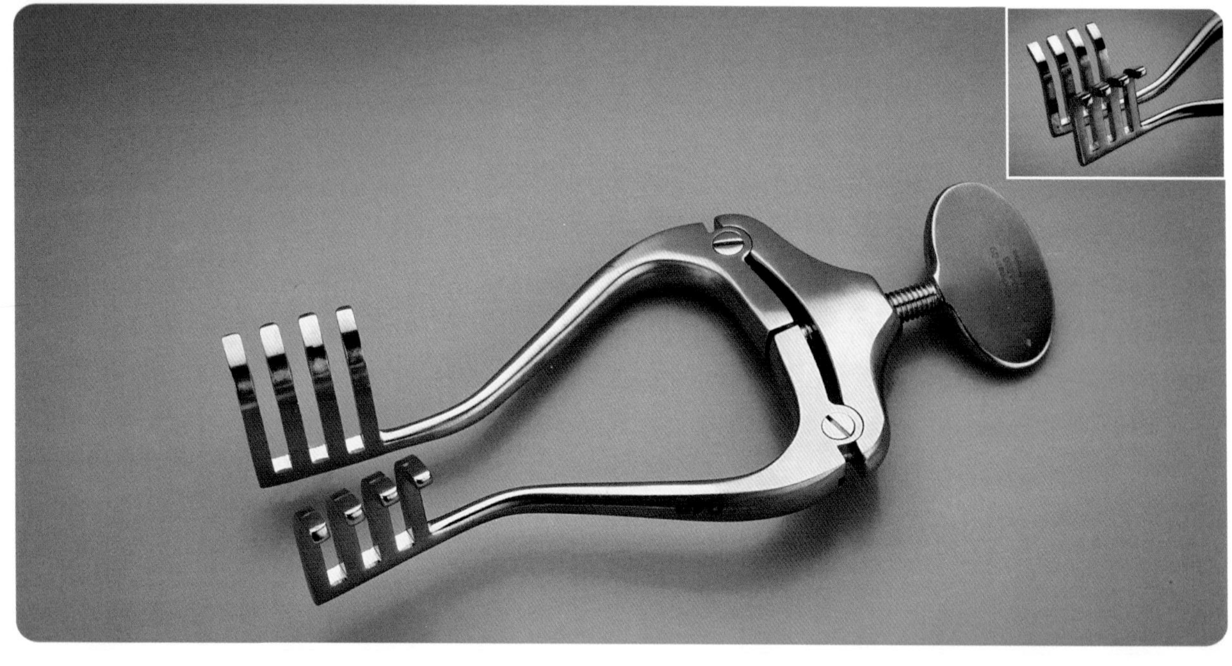

Retractor/Mastoid

USE • To retract tissue during otologic surgery (self-retaining)

VARIETIES • Blunt; 3 × 3 or 4 × 4 prongs

ALSO KNOWN AS • Allport retractor, Gifford retractor, Jansen retractor

210

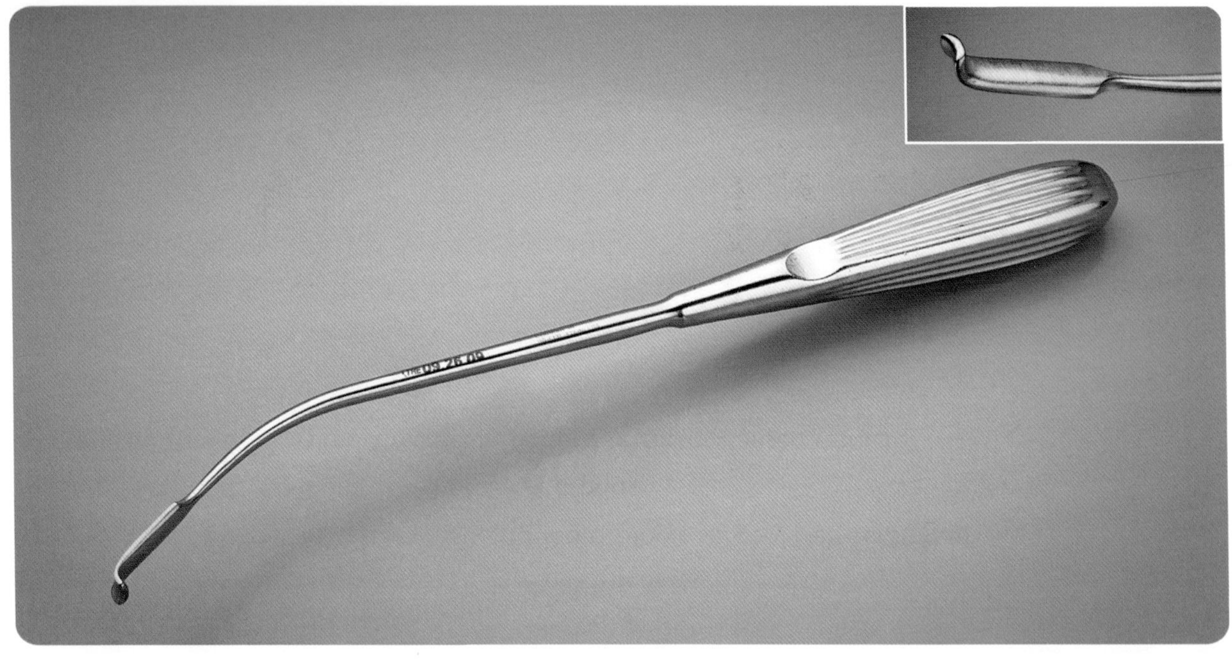

Retractor/Nerve Root

USE • To retract nerve roots during spinal surgery

VARIETIES • Straight or angled; 11 × 13 mm blade

ALSO KNOWN AS • Cushing retractor, Love retractor, Scoville retractor

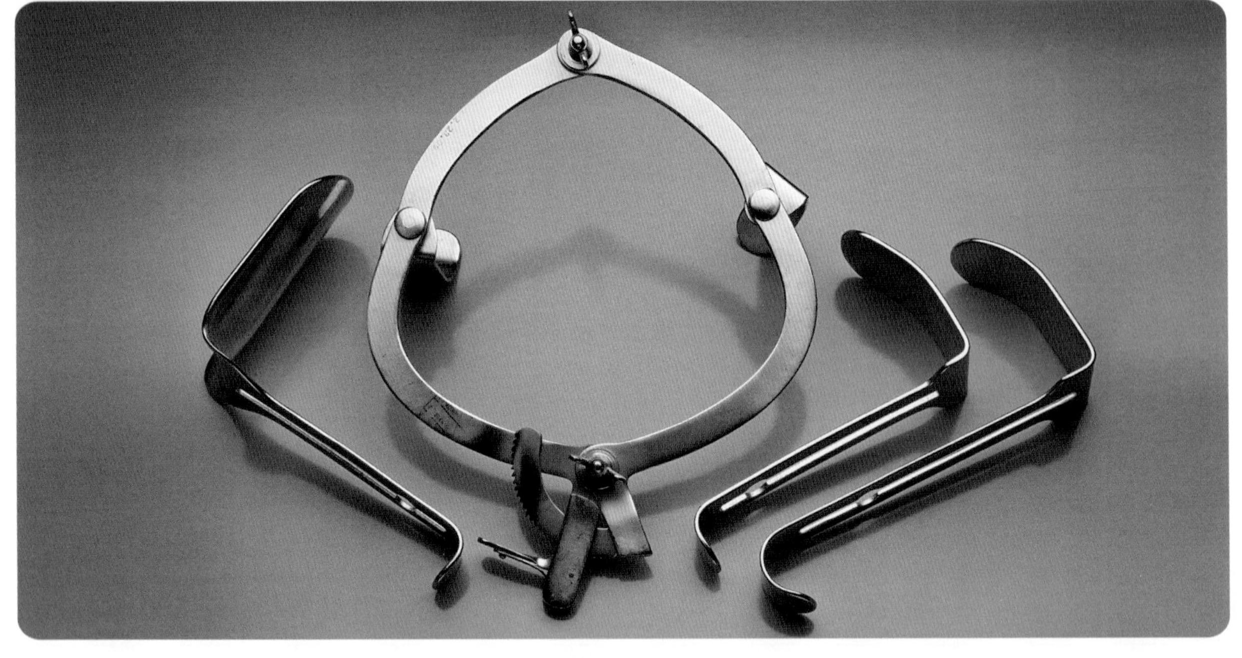

Retractor/O'Connor-O'Sullivan

USE • To retract abdominal wall during intraabdominal or pelvic surgery (self-retaining)

VARIETIES • Attached lateral blades; three interchangeable blades: one large and two small sizes

ALSO KNOWN AS • Gyn retractor

214

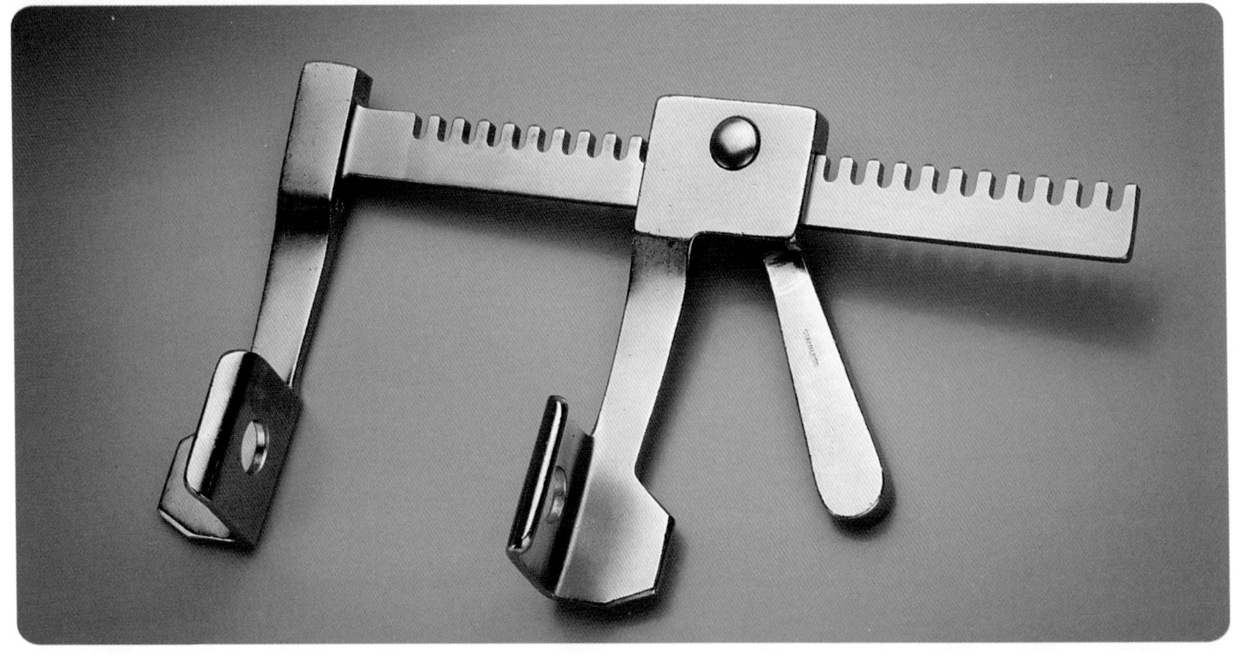

Retractor/Rib

USE
- To retract rib and sternum during thoracic surgery, including open heart surgery (self-retaining)

VARIETIES
- Pediatric and adult sizes

ALSO KNOWN AS
- Burford retractor, chest retractor, Cooley retractor, Cooley-Merz retractor, DeBakey retractor, Finochietto retractor, Harken retractor, Lemmon retractor, Rienhoff-Finochietto retractor, rib spreader, Tuffier retractor, Wilson retractor

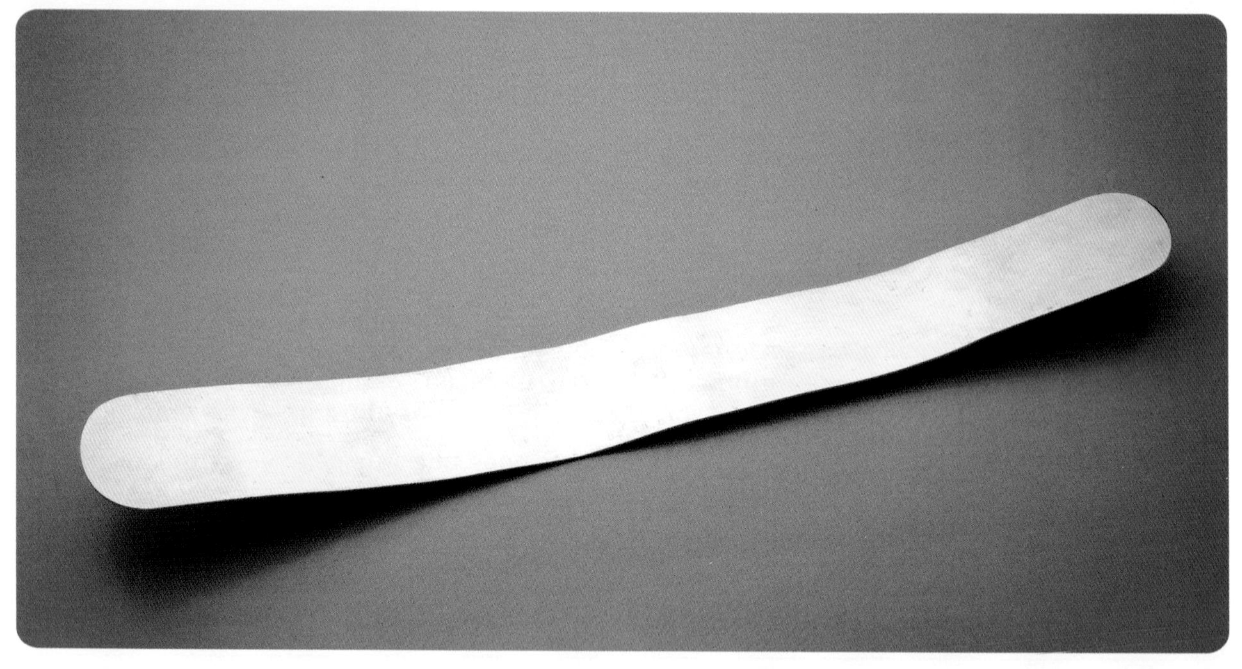

Retractor/Ribbon

USE • To protect soft tissue during dissection; to aid in blunt retraction of bowel and malleable retraction of soft tissue around bone

VARIETIES • Various lengths and widths; malleable

ALSO KNOWN AS • Malleable retractor

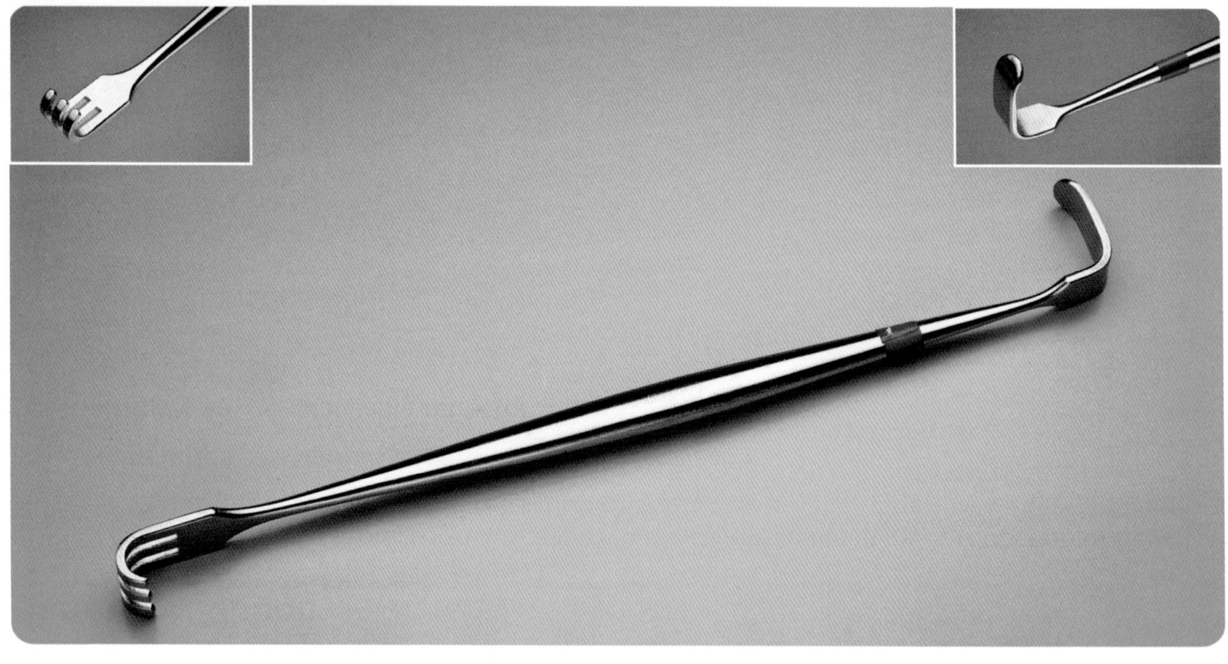

Retractor/Senn

USE • To maintain exposure during superficial plastic surgery or hand surgery

VARIETIES • Double-ended; sharp or blunt prongs

ALSO KNOWN AS • Small rake

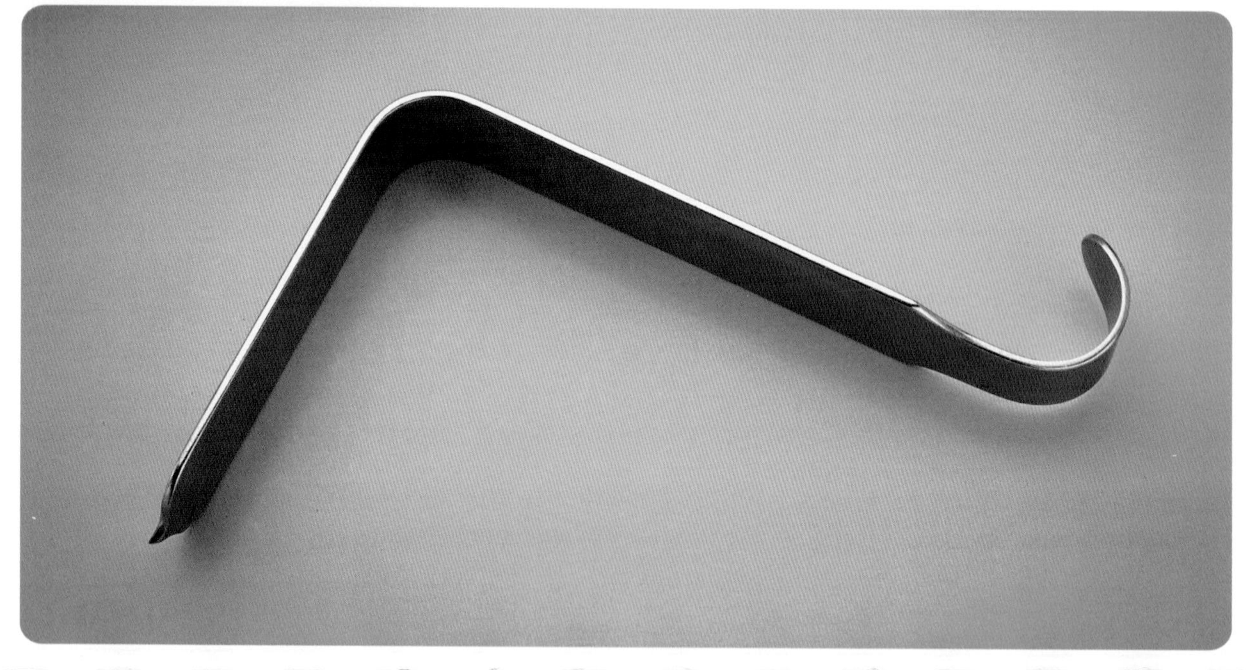

Retractor/Taylor

USE • To maintain spinal retraction during laminectomy; to use for retraction during shoulder surgery (handheld) and hip surgery

VARIETIES • Small or large blades; various lengths

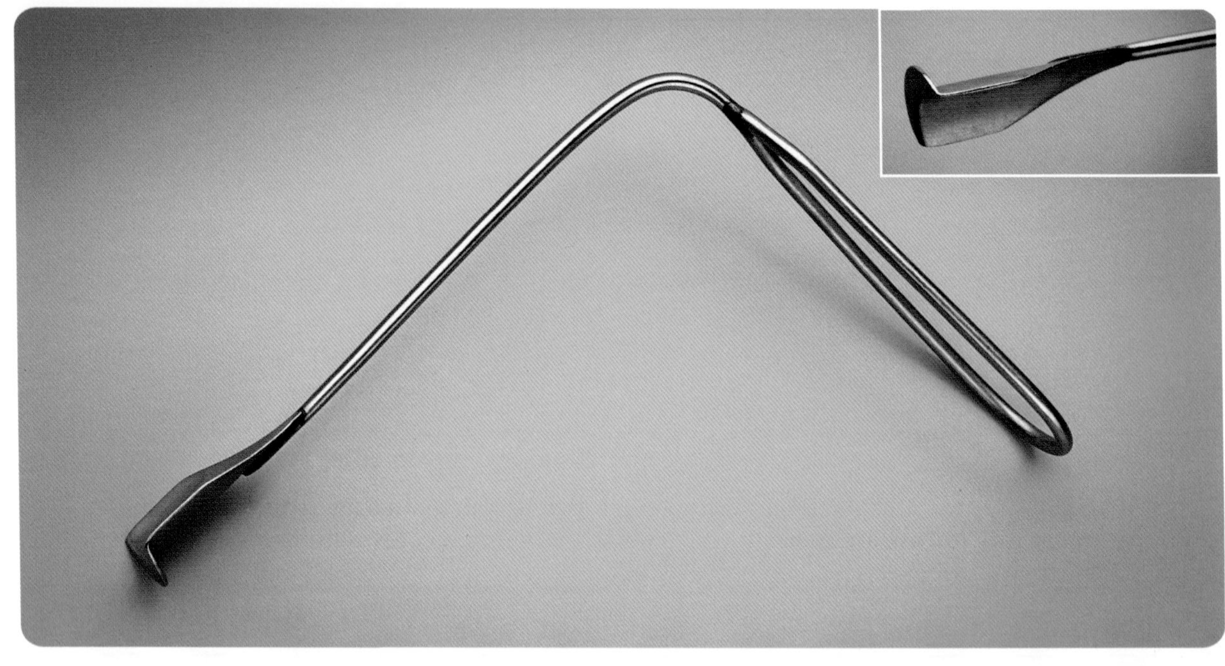

Retractor/Uvula

USE • To retract the posterior soft palate during intraoral procedures

VARIETIES • 8 inches long; grooved blade with 5 mm lip

ALSO KNOWN AS • Brown retractor, Lothrop uvula retractor

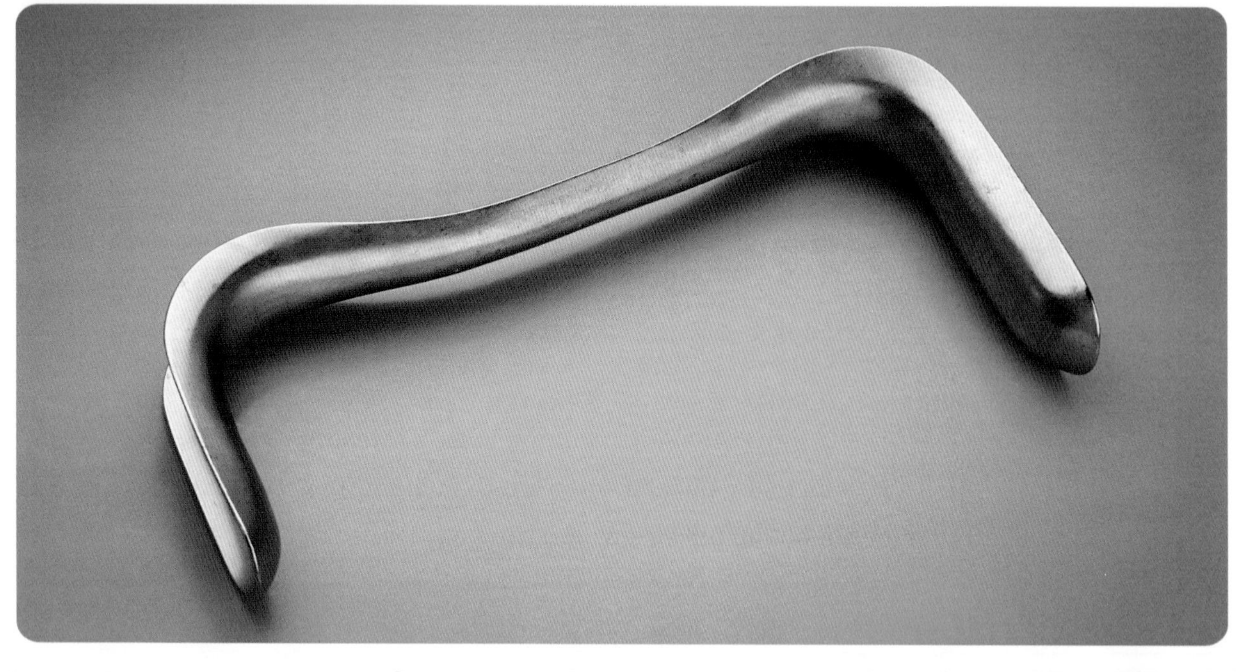

Retractor/Vaginal, Sims

USE • To retract the vaginal wall; to provide exposure during vaginal and transvaginal surgery (handheld)

VARIETIES • Various blade widths and sizes; double-ended

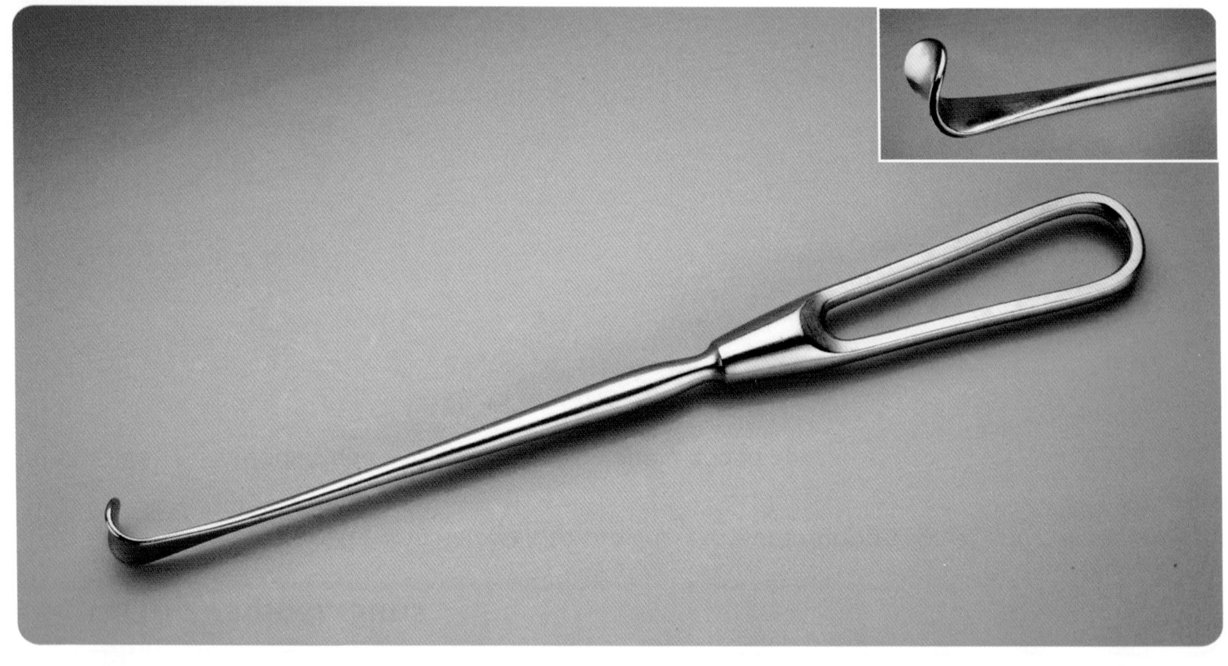

Retractor/Vein

USE	• To retract vessels
VARIETIES	• Plain edge; fenestrated blade; straight with smooth, curved end
ALSO KNOWN AS	• Cushing retractor, Sachs retractor

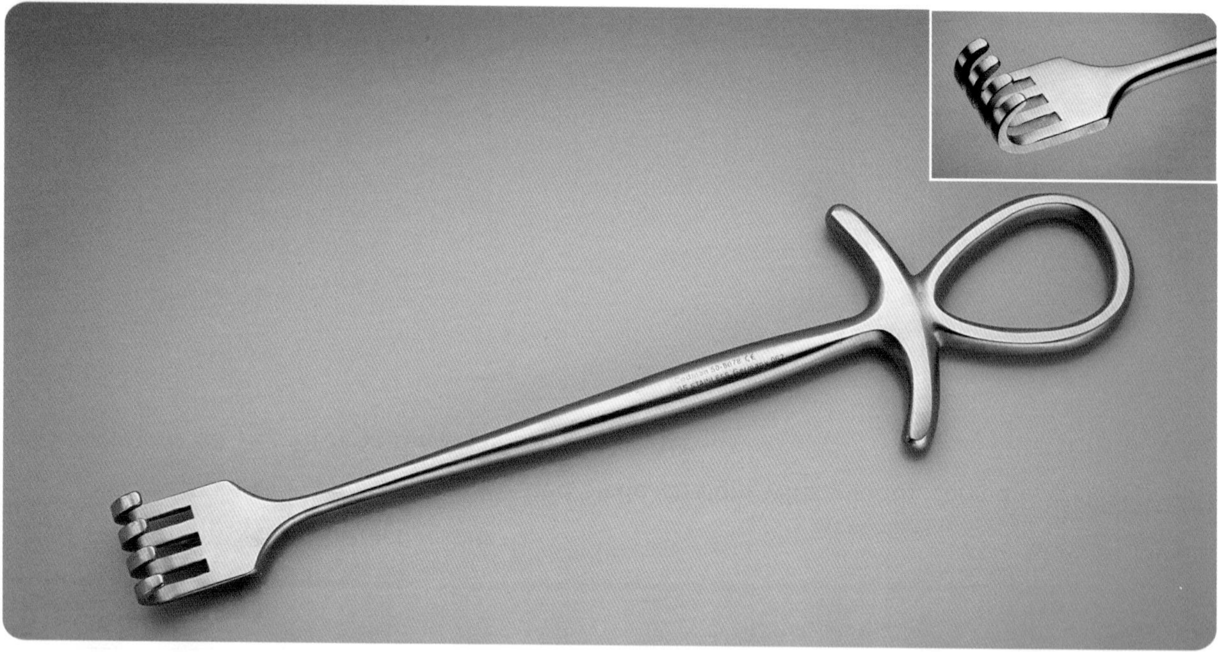

Retractor/Volkmann

USE • To retract superficial tissue (handheld)

VARIETIES • Blunt or sharp; two to six prongs

ALSO KNOWN AS • Rakes

230

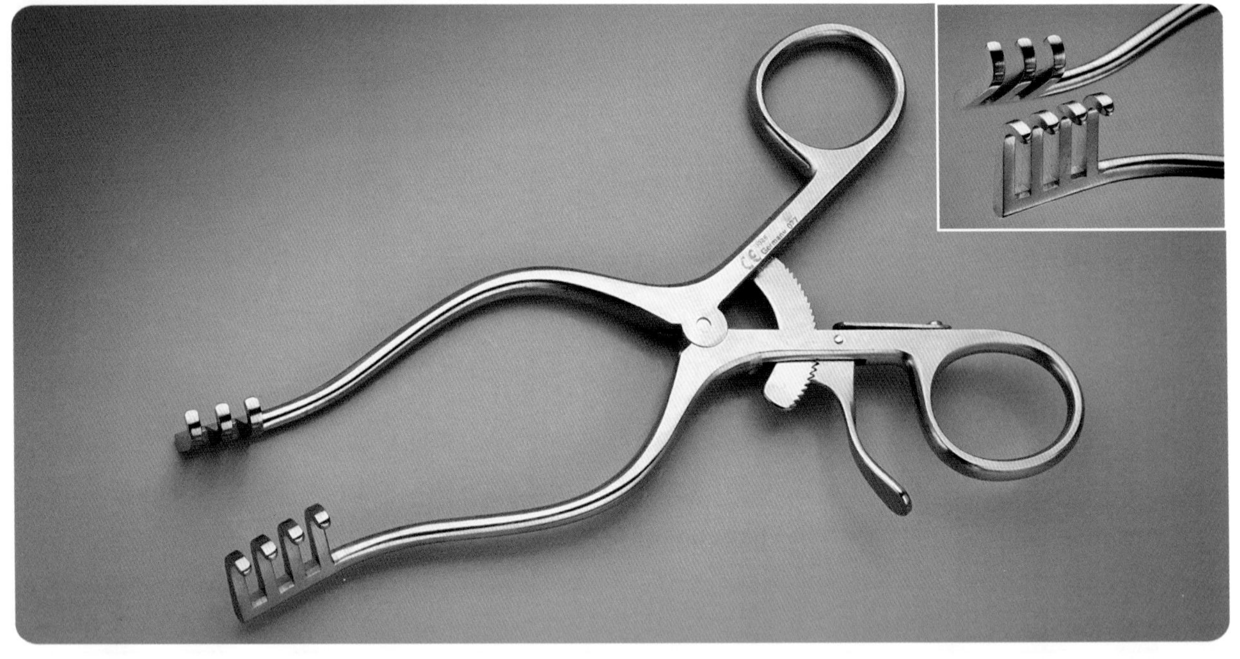

Retractor/Weitlaner

USE • To maintain wound exposure (self-retaining)

VARIETIES • Sharp or blunt jaws; 2 × 3 or 3 × 4 teeth; short to long

ALSO KNOWN AS • Self-retaining retractor

232

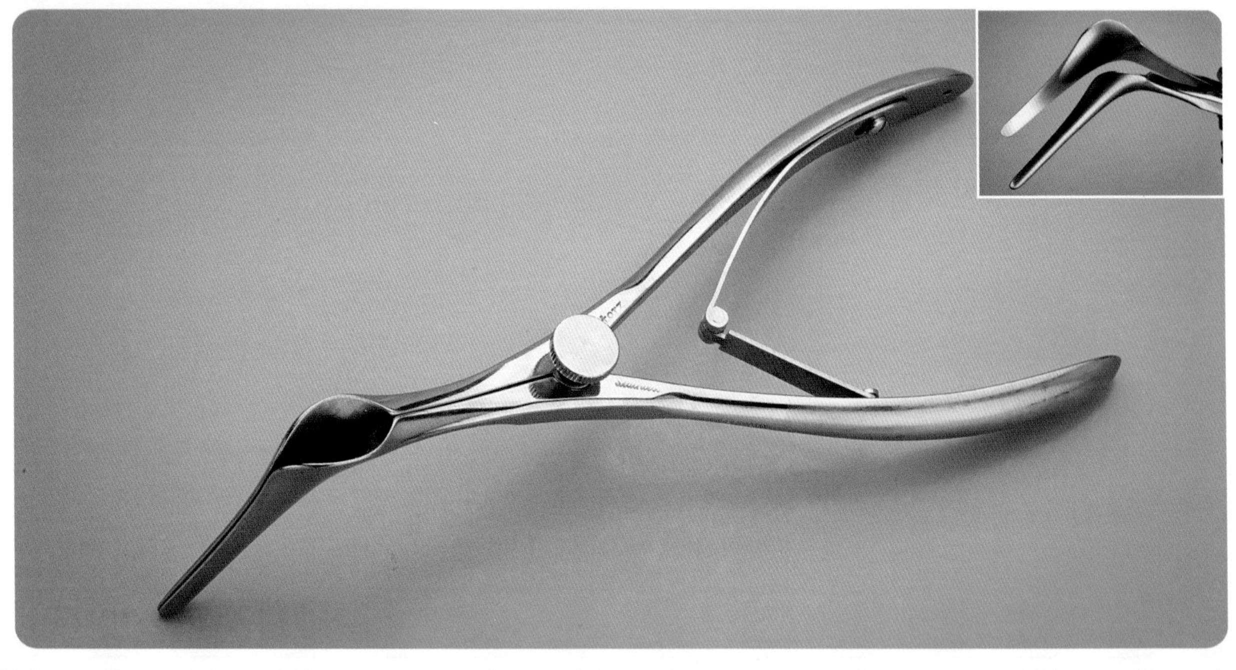

Speculum/Nasal

USE • To visualize intranasal cavity

VARIETIES • Small, medium, large, or extra large sizes

ALSO KNOWN AS • Beckman-Colver speculum, Cottle speculum, Halle-Tieck speculum, Ingals speculum, Killian speculum, Lillie speculum, Merz speculum, Sonnenschein speculum, Tieck speculum, Vienna speculum

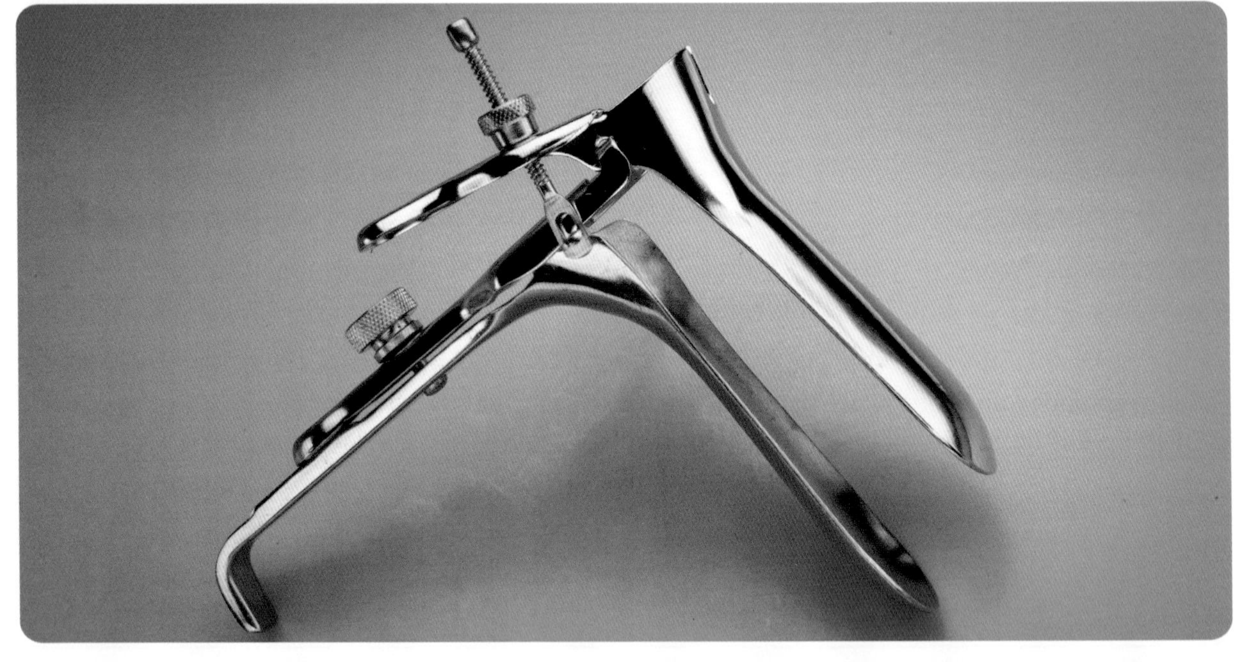

Speculum/Vaginal, Graves

USE • To retract the vaginal wall during vaginal or transvaginal surgery (self-retaining)

VARIETIES • Small, medium, or large blades; stainless steel or disposable plastic

ALSO KNOWN AS • Duckbill speculum, Pederson vaginal speculum, Trélat vaginal speculum

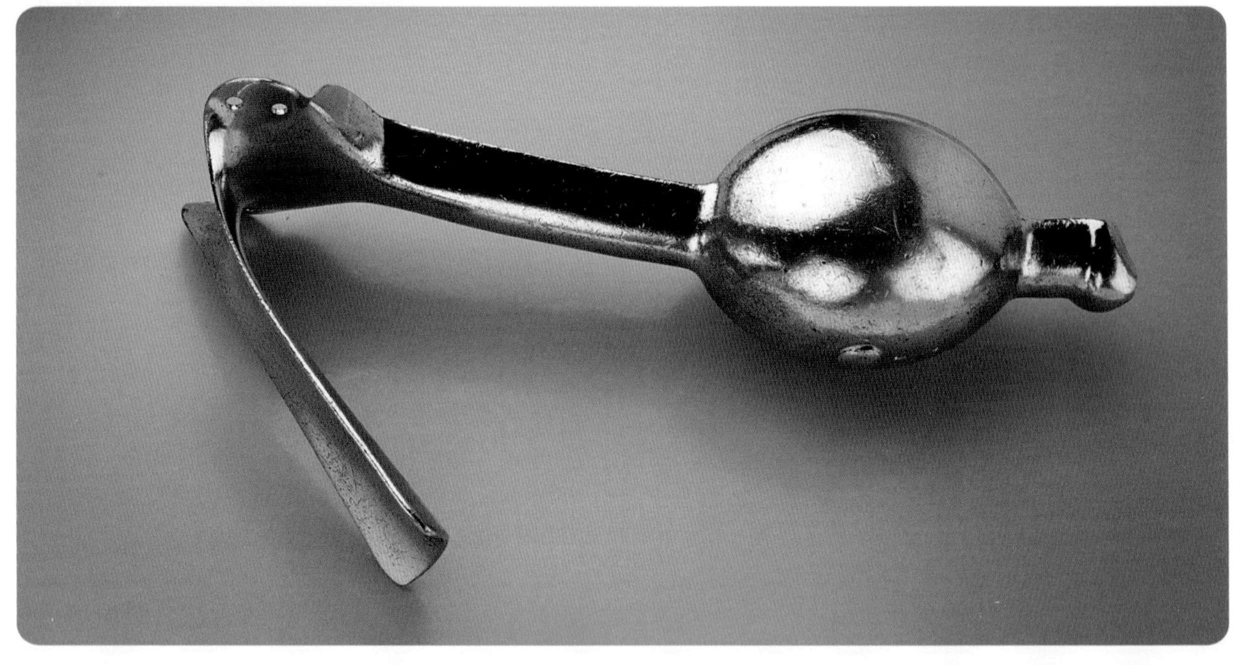

Speculum/Vaginal, Weighted

USE • To retract the posterior vaginal wall during vaginal procedures

VARIETIES • 2¼ or 3 pounds; shallow or deep; narrow or wide; chrome-plated or stainless steel

ALSO KNOWN AS • Auvard speculum, Garrigue speculum, Picot speculum

CHAPTER 5

Suture Devices/Needle Holders

Suture devices are surgical instruments used to hold and pass suture needles through tissue. They are also used to close wounds.

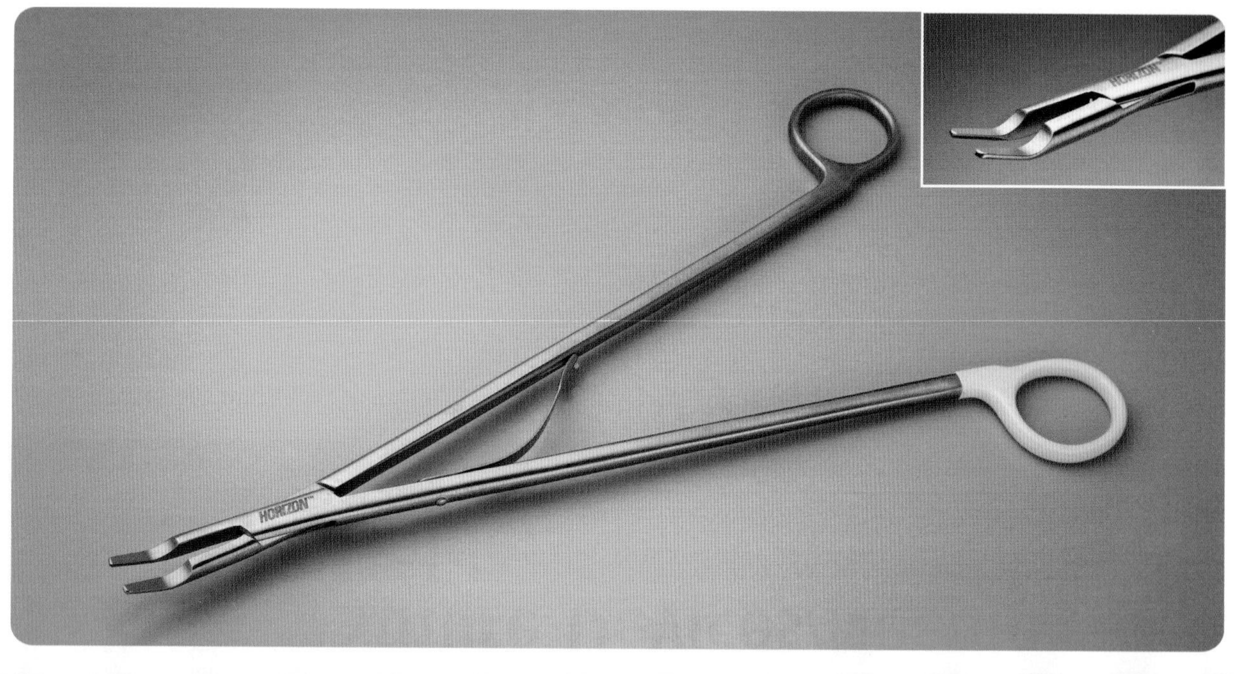
HORIZON™
HORIZON™

Clip Applier/Ligating

USE • To apply vessel ligating clips

VARIETIES • Small, medium, large, or extra large clips; curved or right-angled jaws; long or short handles; handles sometimes color-coded to match ligating clip cartridges

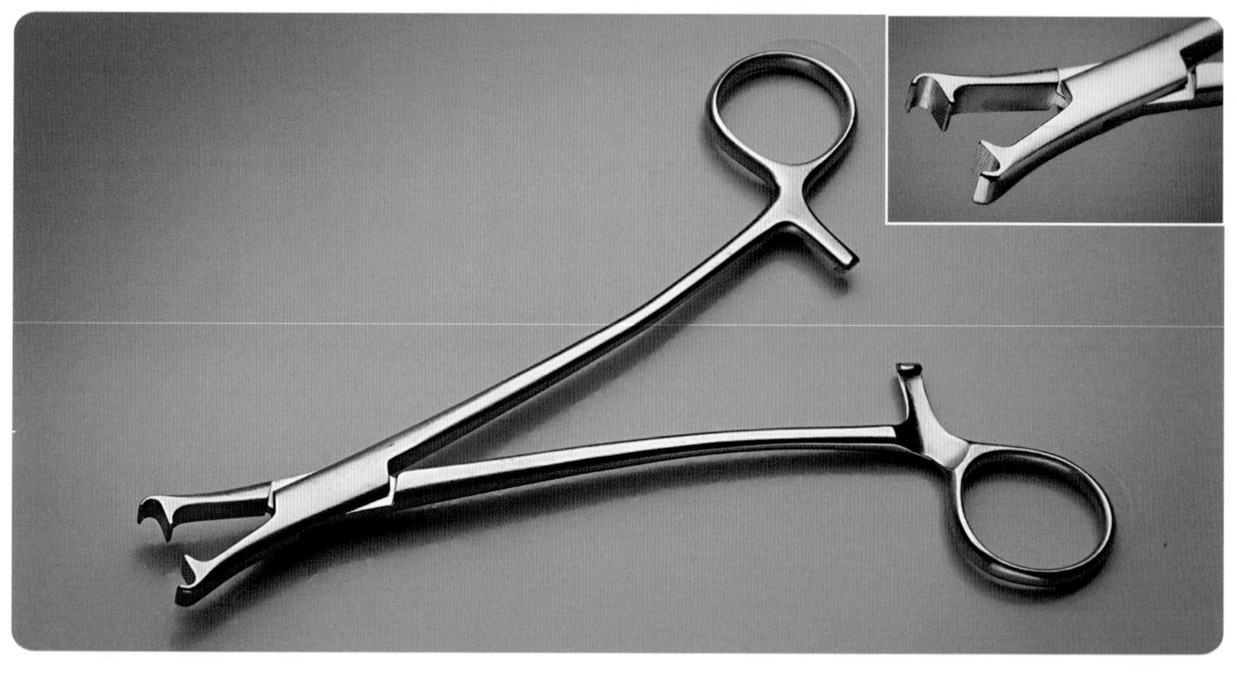

Clip Applier/Raney

USE • To apply a hemostatic clip (disposable) to scalp incision edges during craniotomy, craniofacial surgery, or plastic surgery (e.g., brow lift)

VARIETIES • One size

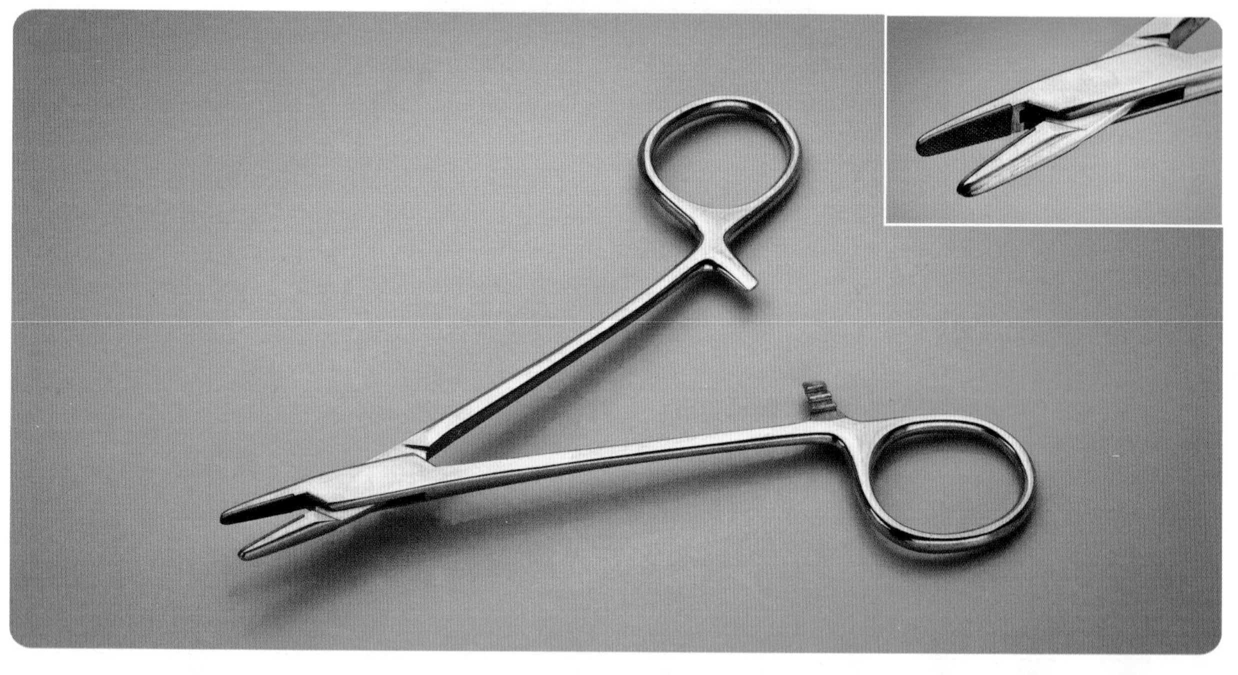

Needle Holder/Baumgartner

USE • To hold heavy plastic surgery needles

VARIETIES • One standard size (5 inches); recommended for suture sizes 2-0 and larger

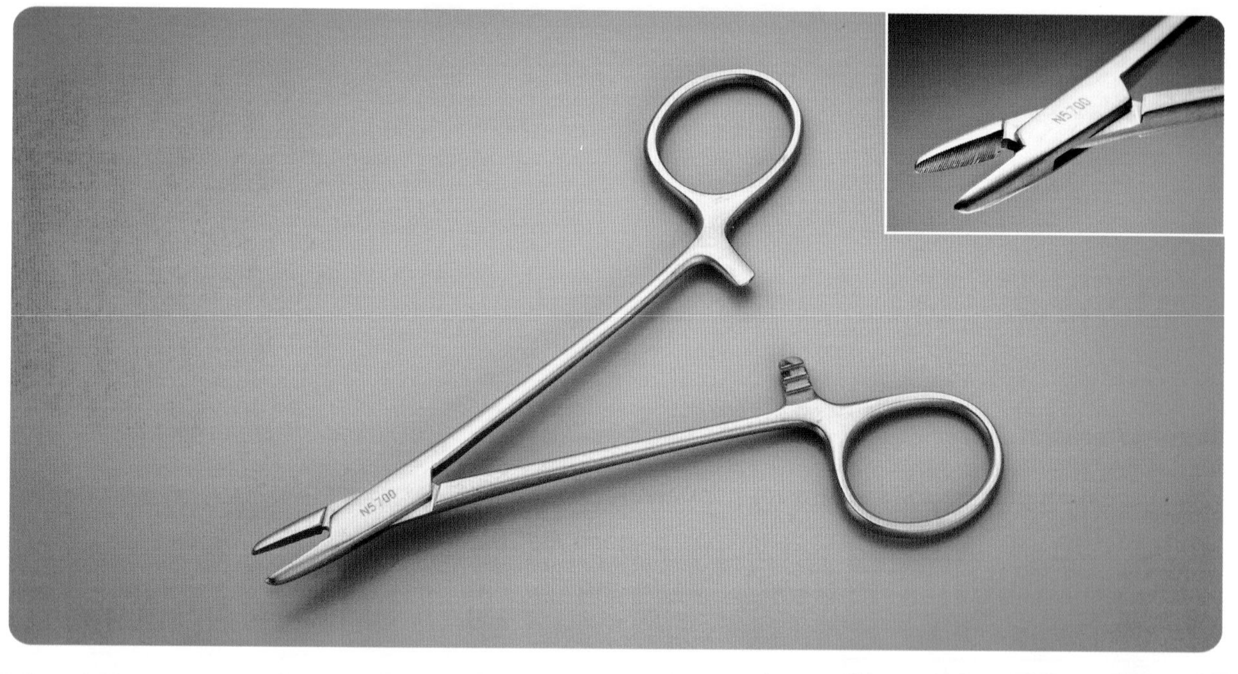
N5700
N5700

Needle Holder/Brown

USE • To apply sutures in superficial tissue (e.g., plastic surgery)

VARIETIES • 5 to 6¾ inches long

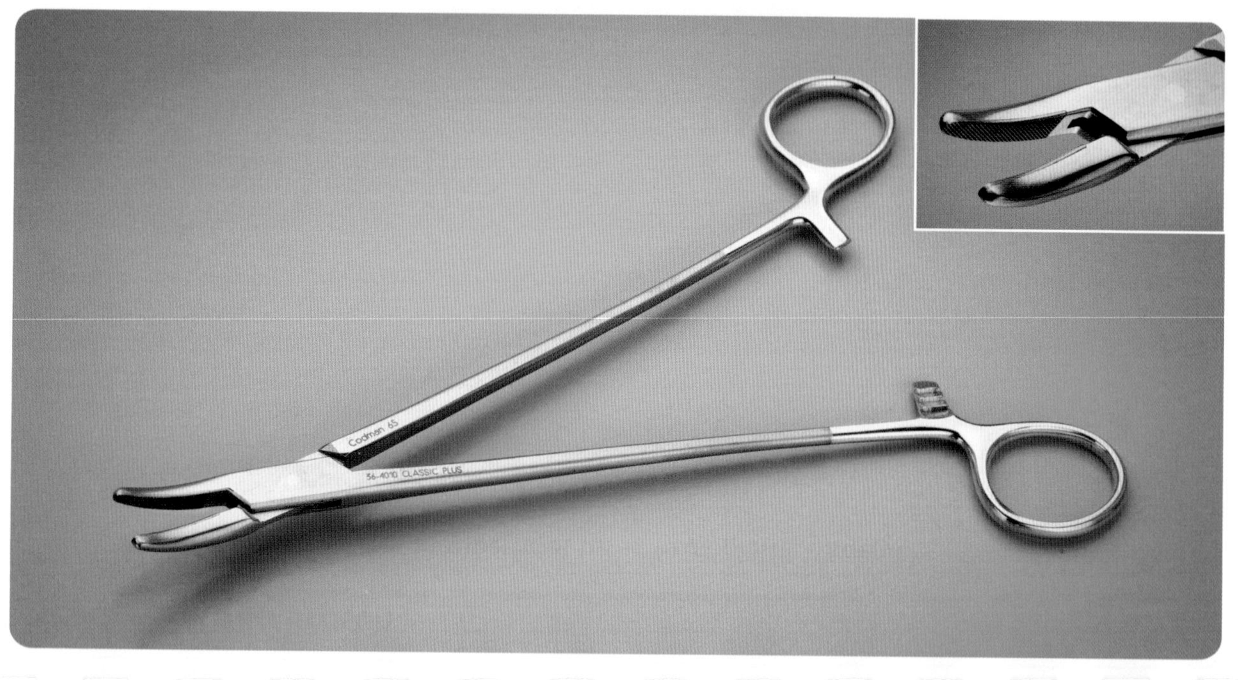
Codman 65
56-4010 CLASSIC PLUS

Needle Holder/Heaney

USE • To hold suture needles during procedures in which an angled tip facilitates proper needle placement (e.g., vaginal hysterectomy)

VARIETIES • Angled jaw; 8 ¼ inches long

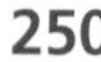

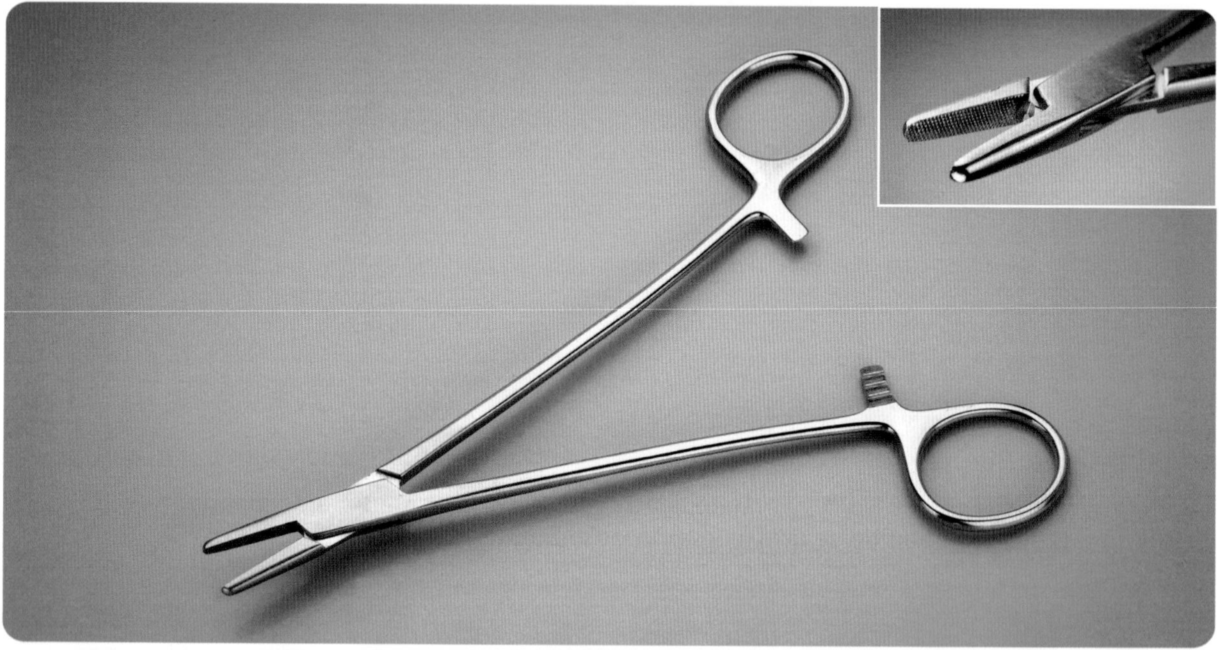

250

Needle Holder/Mayo-Hegar

USE • To apply heavy sutures (e.g., during cardiothoracic surgery); also widely used in general surgery

VARIETIES • 6 ¼ to 12 inches long; recommended for suture sizes 2-0 and larger

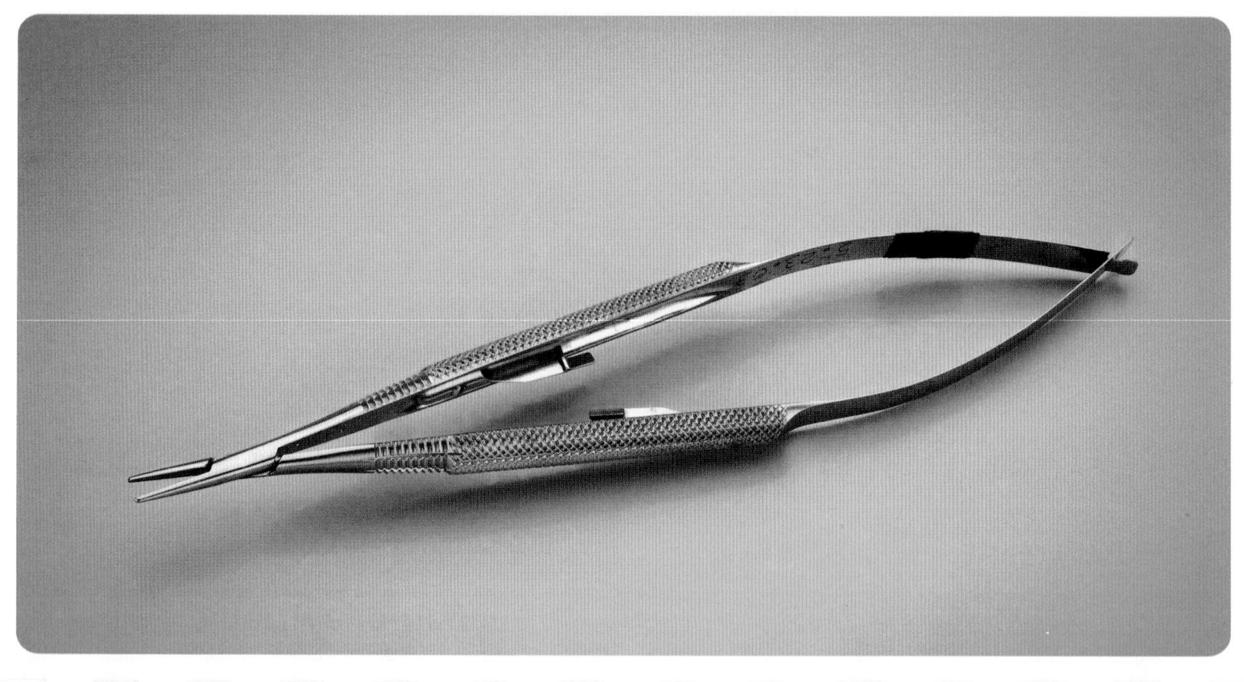

Needle Holder/Microvascular

USE • To hold fine, microvascular needles

VARIETIES • With or without catch; straight or curved; serrated or smooth jaws; 5¾ to 7 inches long; used with fine sutures, sizes 8-0 through 11-0

ALSO KNOWN AS • Castroviejo needle holder

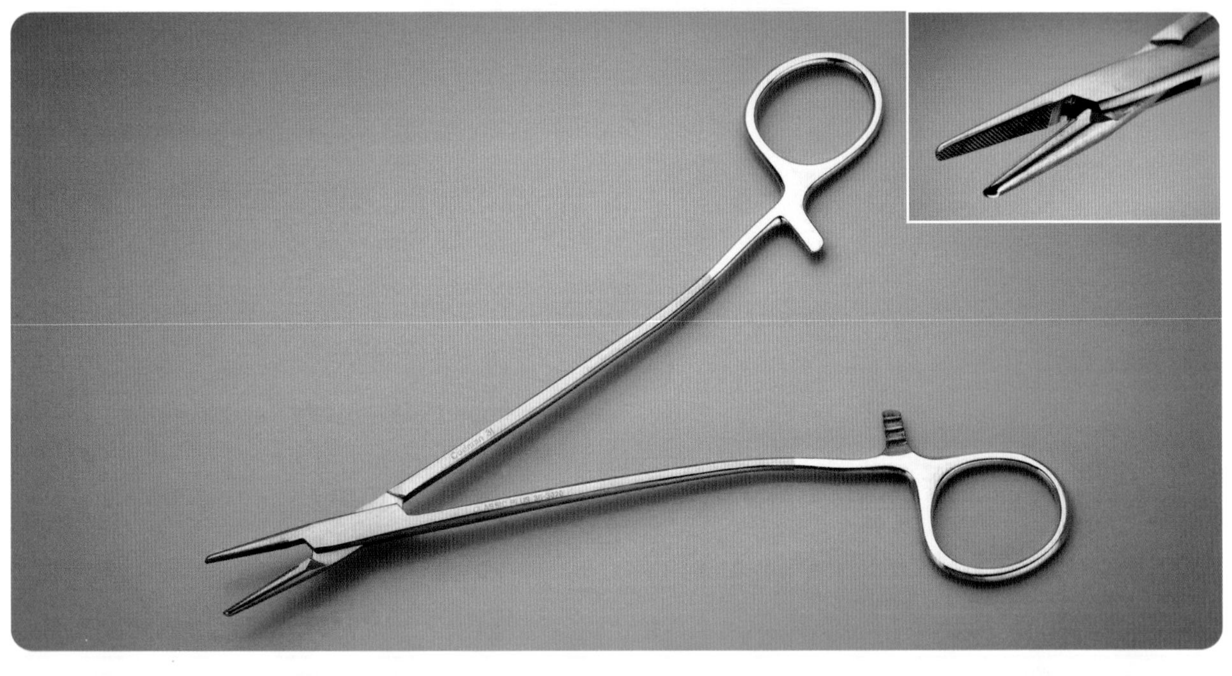

Needle Holder/Sarot

USE • To hold fine, delicate needles (e.g., cardiovascular needles)

VARIETIES • 7 or 10 ½ inches long; recommended for suture sizes 4-0 to 2

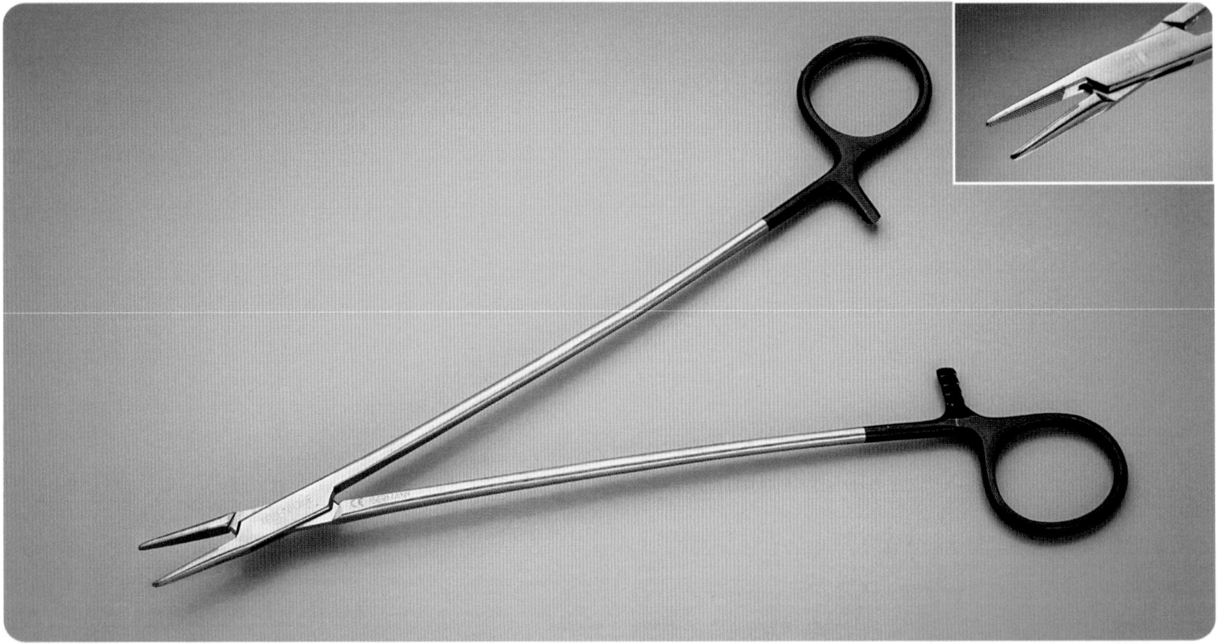

256

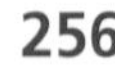

Needle Holder/Vascular

USE • To hold fine, delicate needles (e.g., cardiovascular needles)

VARIETIES • Smooth jaw inserts; 6, 6¾, or 8 inches long

CHAPTER 6

Suction Tips

Suction tips are used to remove blood and other fluids from a surgical or operative field to provide better visualization.

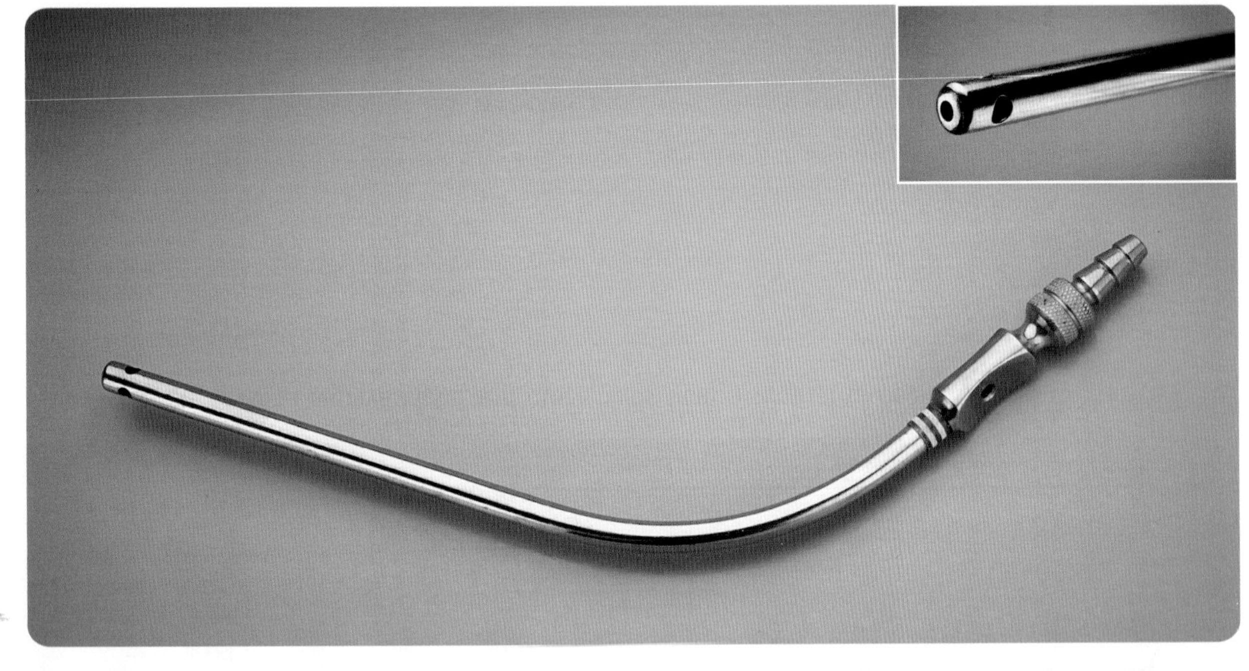

Suction Tip/Abdominal

USE
- To evacuate a fluid-filled cavity or to prevent accumulation of fluid (e.g., in the abdominal cavity)

VARIETIES
- Long or short tip; stainless steel or disposable plastic

ALSO KNOWN AS
- Ferguson abdominal suction tip

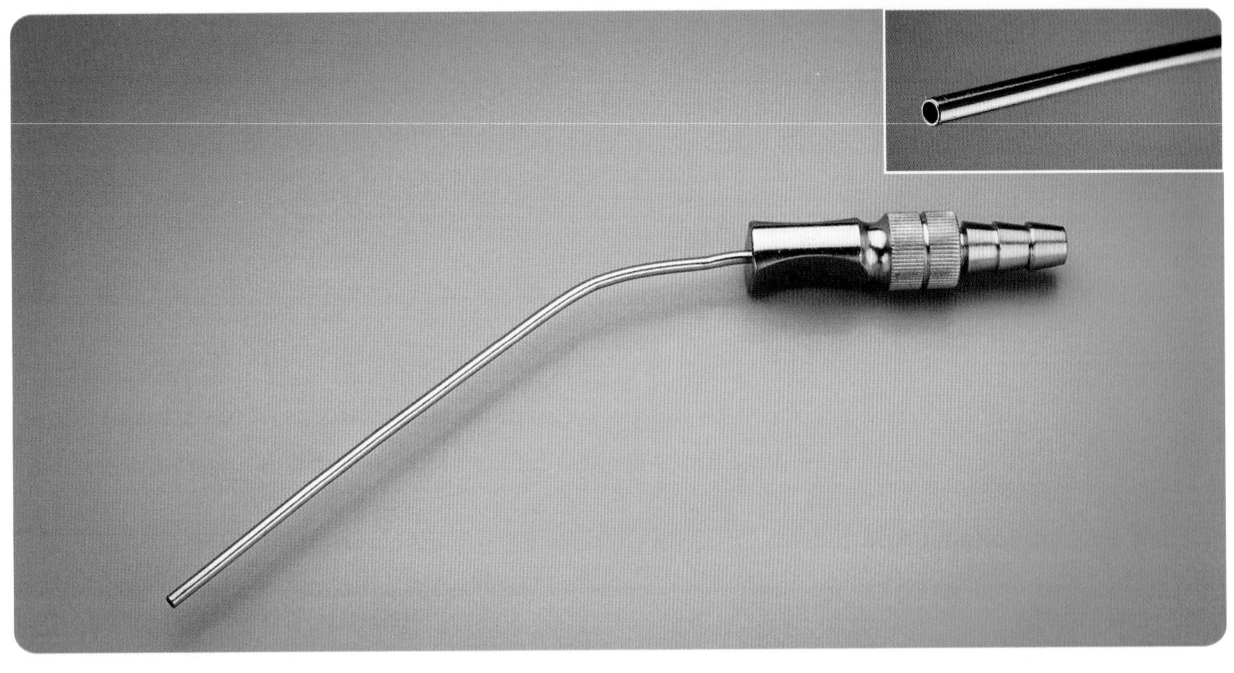

Suction Tip/Frazier

USE • To evacuate small quantities of accumulated fluid (e.g., during plastic or peripheral vascular surgery)

VARIETIES • Angled or straight; short or long tip (for deeper suctioning); metal or disposable; 6 to 16 French diameter

ALSO KNOWN AS • Ferguson-Frazier suction tip

264

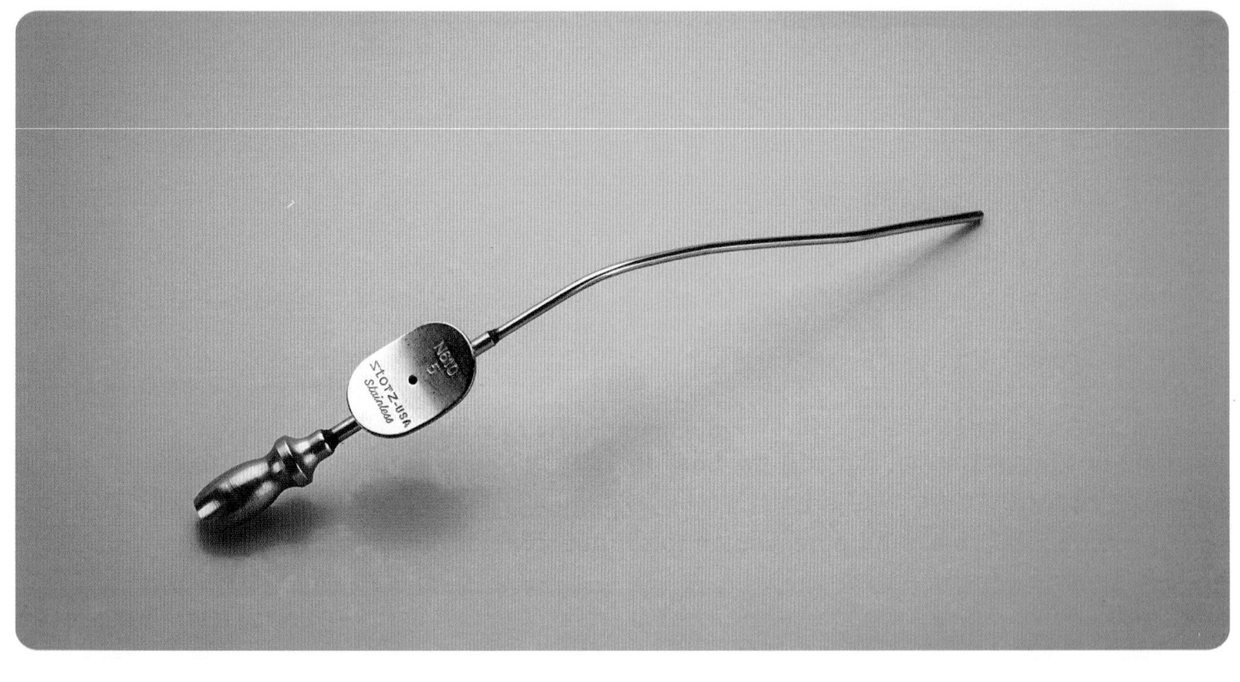

Suction Tip/Plastic

USE • To remove fluids during superficial plastic surgery

VARIETIES • Metal; 3 to 7 French diameter with finger cut off; angled or straight

ALSO KNOWN AS • Baron suction tip

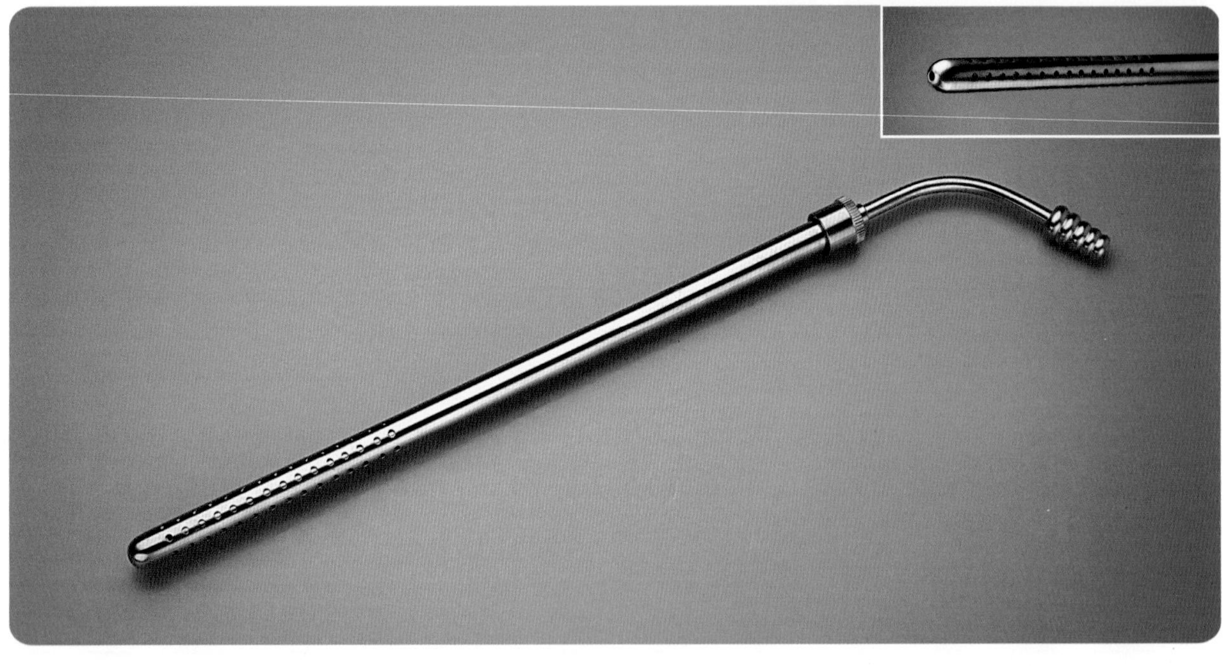

Suction Tip/Poole

USE • To remove ascites or irrigation fluid from abdominal or chest cavity

VARIETIES • Straight or curved; metal or disposable; 23 or 30 French diameter

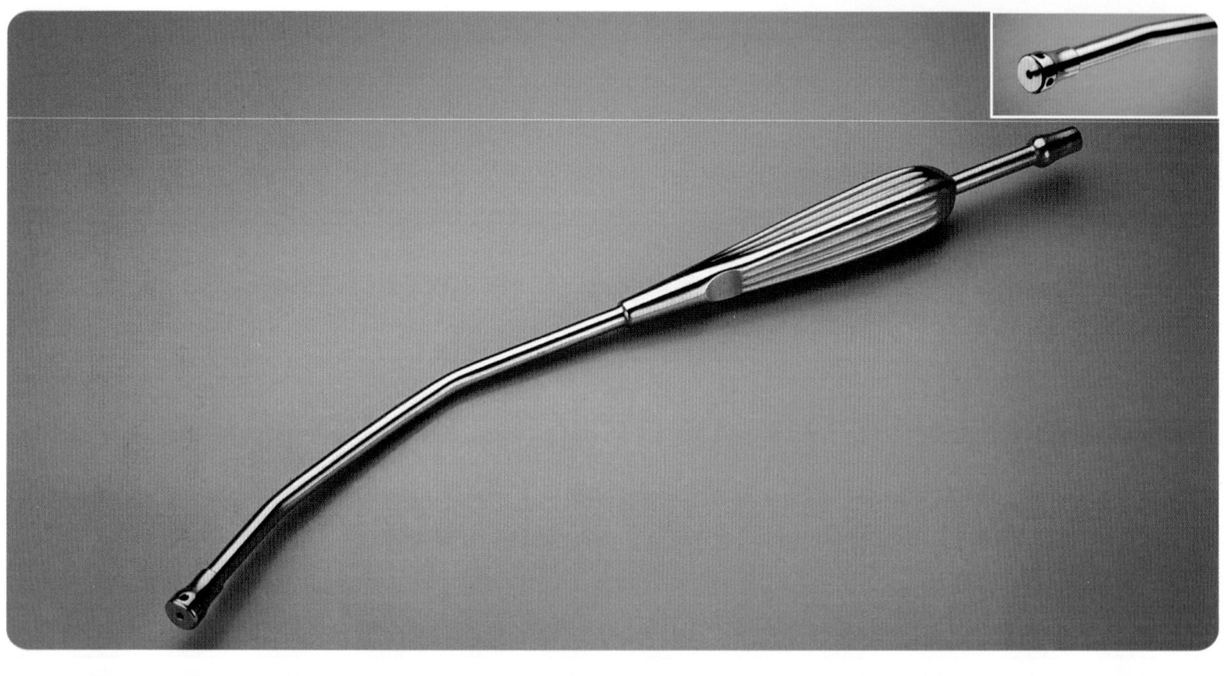

Suction Tip/Yankauer

USE • To remove fluid during intraoral, intraabdominal, or intrathoracic surgical procedures

VARIETIES • Metal or disposable; with or without control valve; pediatric and adult sizes

ALSO KNOWN AS • Tonsil suction tip

CHAPTER 7

Dilators/Probes

Dilators are used to enlarge or expand the size of an opening. They provide access to narrow passages or incisions.

272

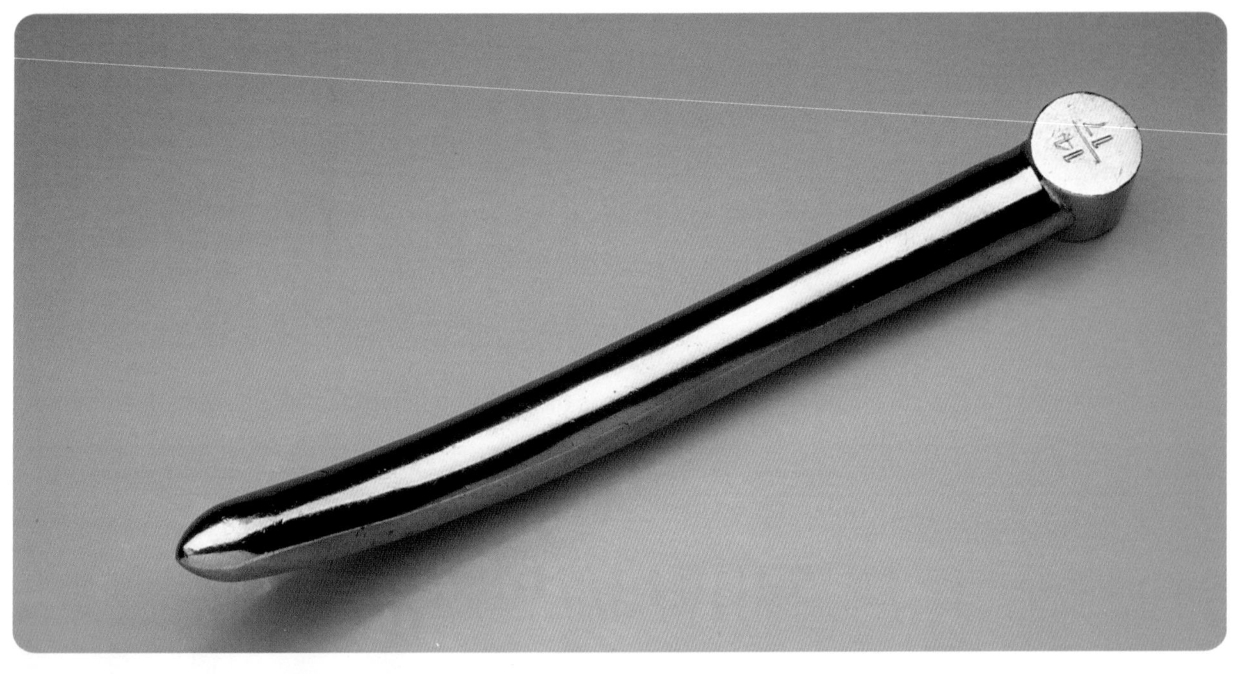

Dilator/Hawkins

USE • To dilate the cervix transvaginally for intrauterine surgery

VARIETIES • Graduated sizes, 8 to 13 cm

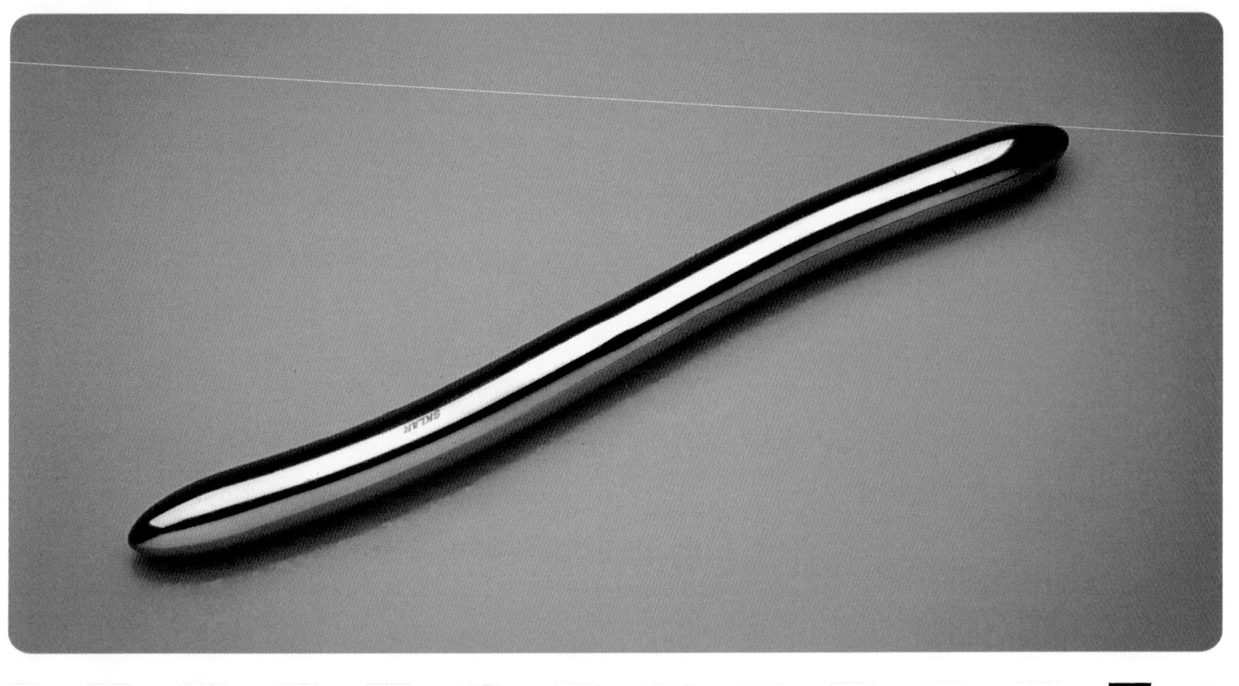
SKLAR

Dilator/Hegar

USE • To dilate the cervix

VARIETIES • Single-ended: Sizes 1–26 mm; 7 inches long

Double-ended: Sizes 3–4 mm to 17–18 mm; 7½ inches long

ALSO KNOWN AS • Cigar dilator

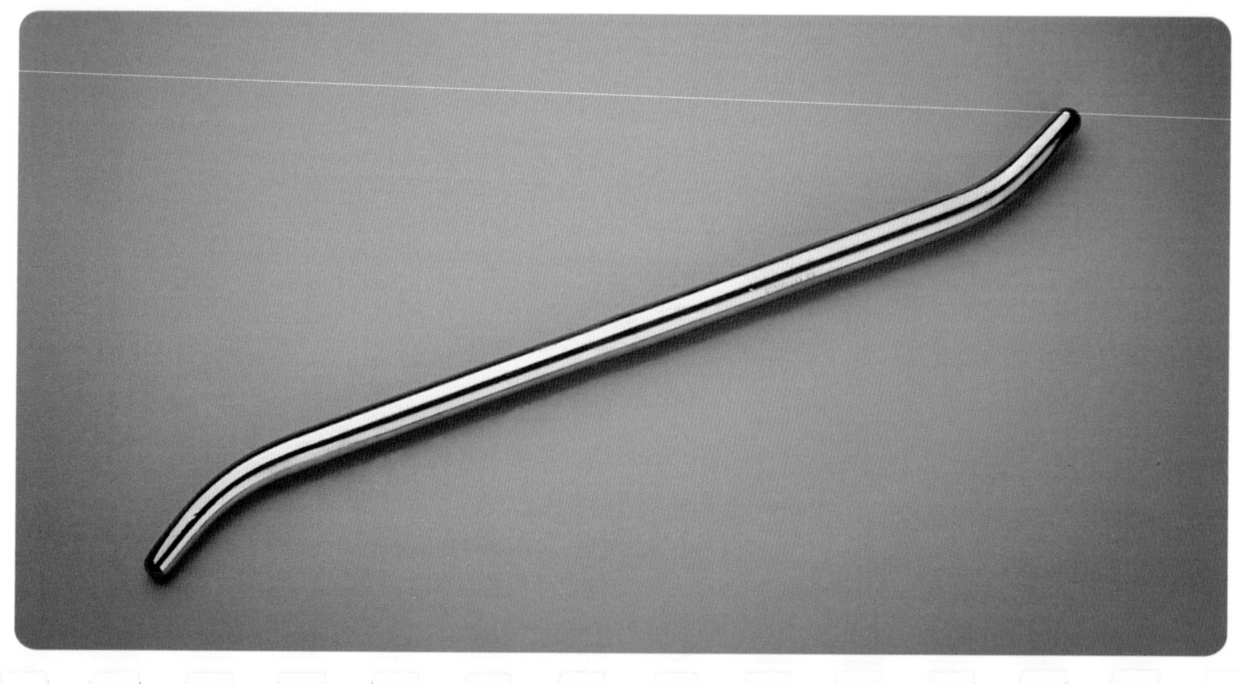

Dilator/Pratt

USE • To dilate the cervix transvaginally

VARIETIES • Double-ended: Sizes 13–15 French diameter to 41–43 French diameter; 11 inches long

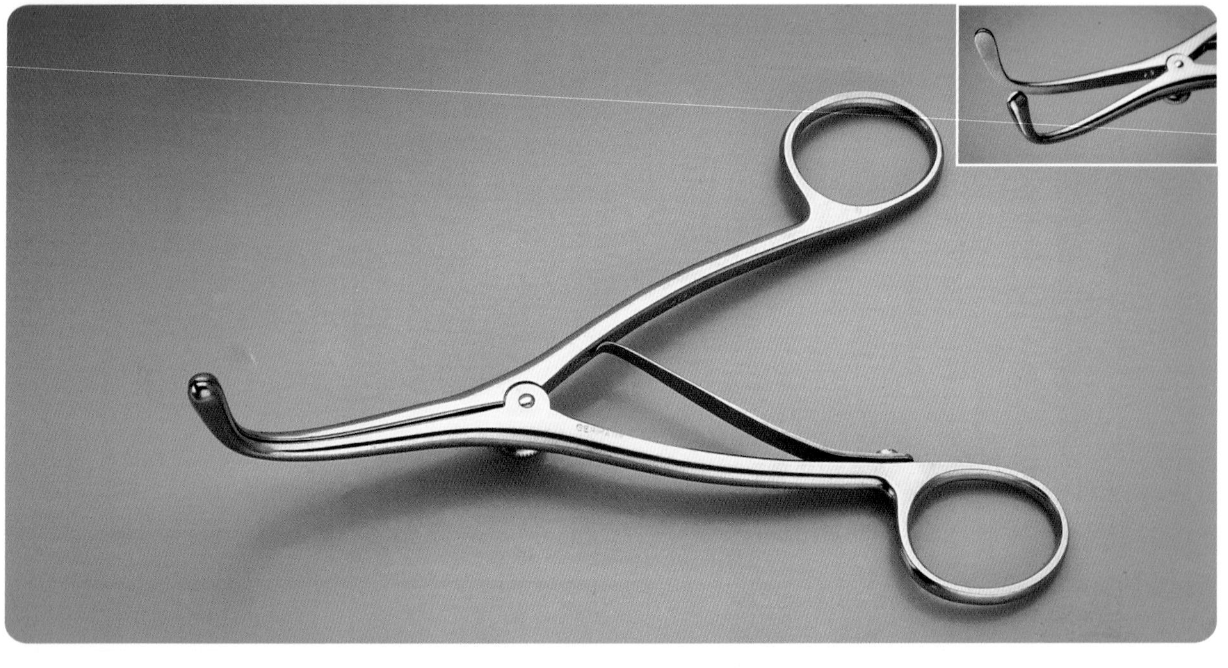

Dilator/Tracheal

USE • To open the trachea during tracheostomy

VARIETIES • Infant, pediatric, and adult sizes; 5 ½ inches

ALSO KNOWN AS • Laborde dilator, Trousseau-Jackson dilator

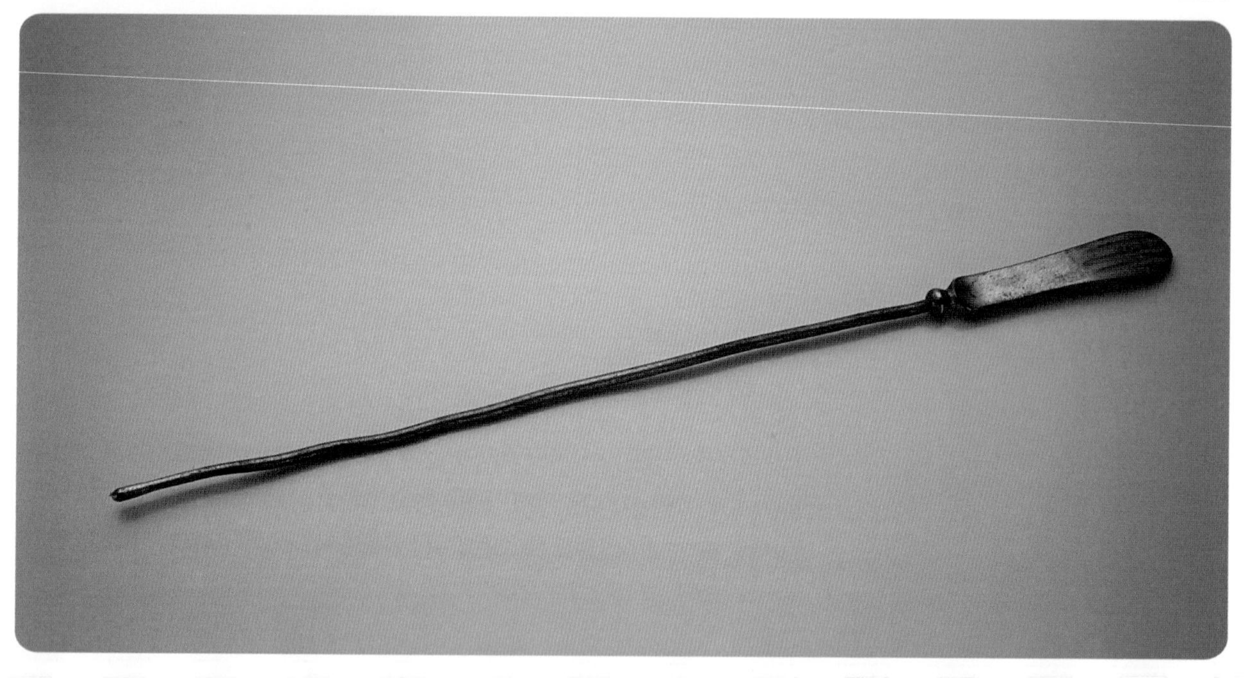

Dilator/Uterine Sound, Sims

USE • Inserted through the cervix to measure the intrauterine cavity depth

VARIETIES • Malleable; graduated in inches or centimeters; 12½ or 13 inches long

ALSO KNOWN AS • Uterine depth gauge

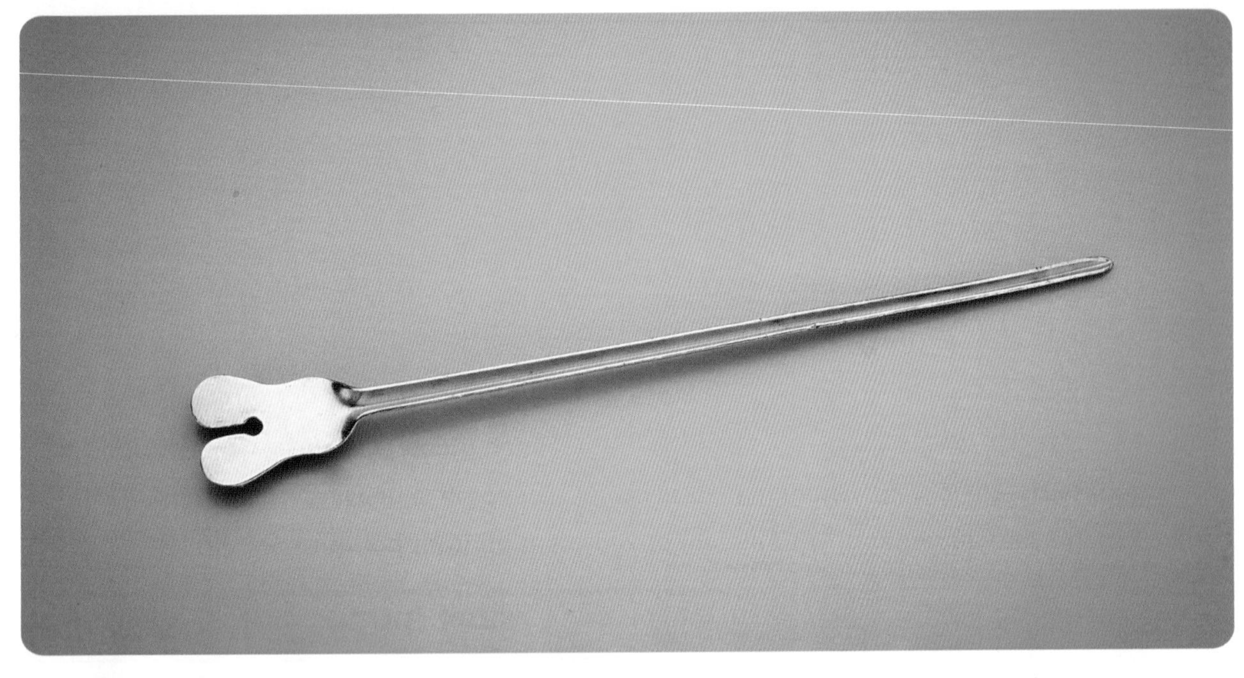

Director/Grooved

USE • To probe vessels during general or vascular surgery; to use in conjunction with a probe to find a fistula tract

VARIETIES • Probe tip or spear end; 4 ½ to 8 inches long; malleable

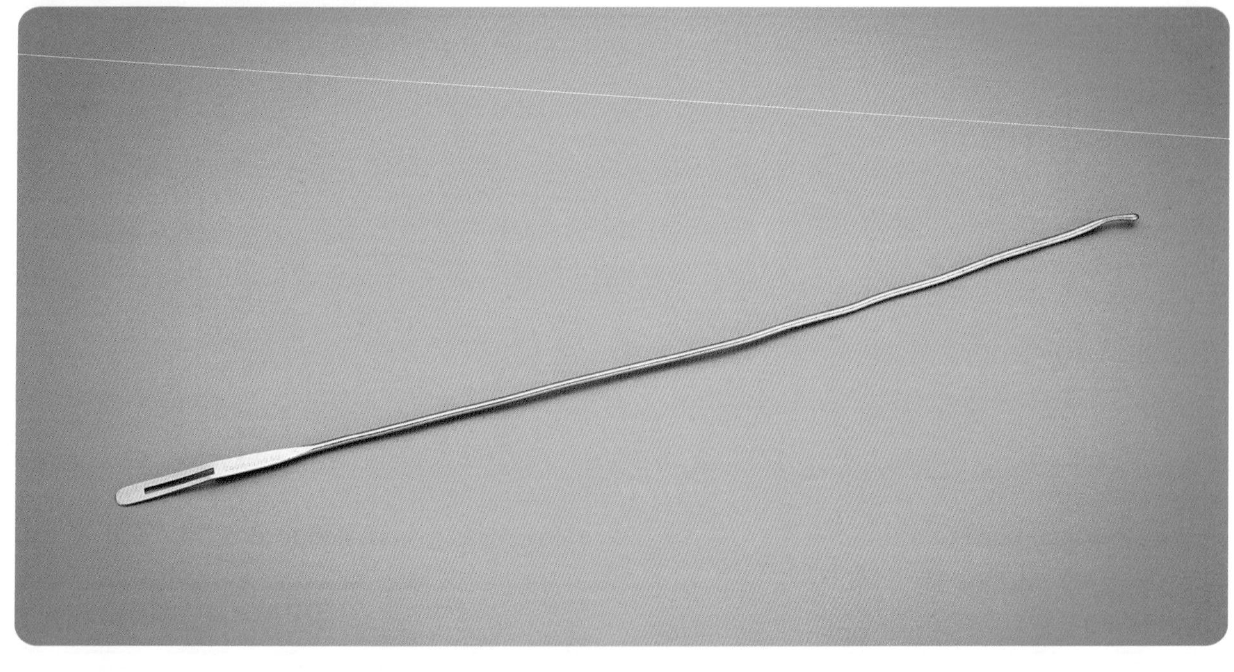

Probe

USE • To gauge depth or direction of a sinus or cavity by inserting it therein; used in conjunction with a groove director

VARIETIES • Stainless steel or sterling silver; double-ended; malleable; various sizes

ALSO KNOWN AS • Buie fistula probe, Desjardins probe, Lacrimal duct probe

CHAPTER 8 Minimally Invasive Surgical Instruments

Minimally invasive surgical (MIS) instruments are long and thin and may be articulated to allow access from a restricted number of trocar ports. These instruments are used for both laparoscopic and robotic surgeries. MIS instruments utilize modern technology to perform most surgical operations through small incisions (less than ½ inch). An MIS procedure typically involves the use of laparoscopic devices and remote control manipulation of instruments with indirect observation of the surgical field. Through an endoscope or similar device, specifically designed instruments permit surgeons to dissect, remove, repair, and reconstruct pathologies through small incisions. MIS instruments are usually graspers, dissectors, and shears. MIS equipment usually includes scopes, cameras, insufflators, light sources, robots, etc.

The current standard of handheld MIS instruments has limitations. Rotation is minimal; it is impossible to achieve fully rotatable wristlike motions (e.g., suturing). Depth perception, which is 2D, is insufficient to facilitate accurate hand-eye coordination. The robotic surgical system is the current solution to those problems and is the next advanced surgical tool associated with minimal invasive surgery. The robotic endoscopic wrist instruments offer greater precision, flexibility, and control than is possible with the standard laparoscopic instruments.

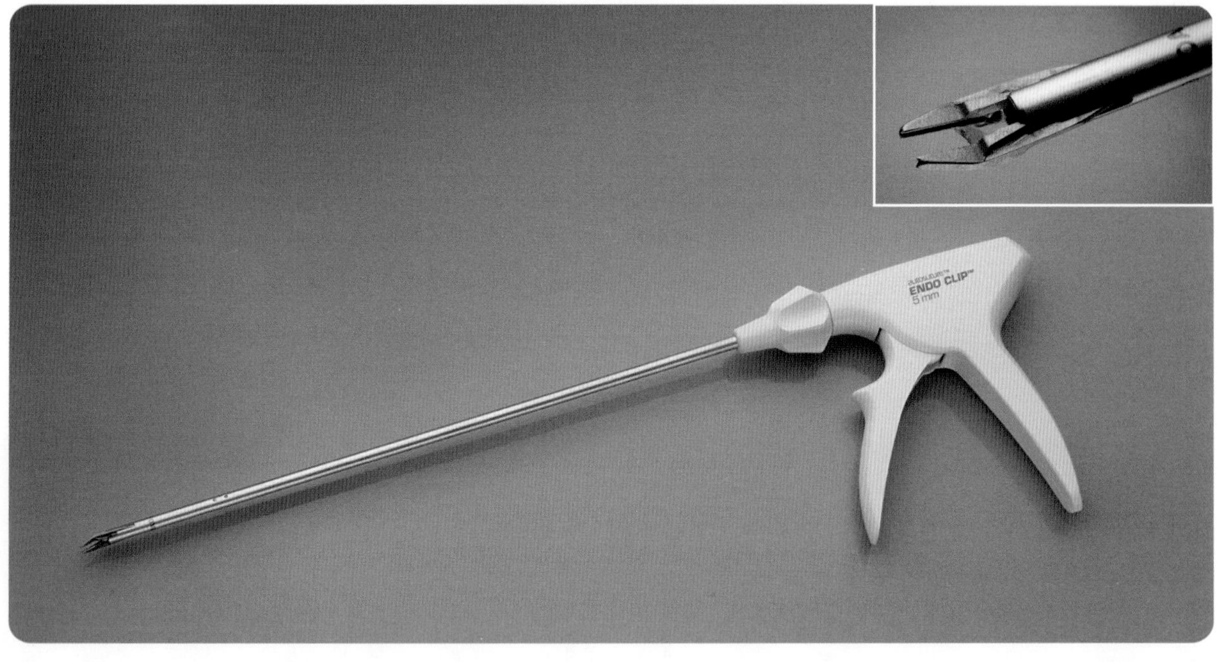
ENDO CLIP™
5 mm

Clip Applier/Endoscopic

USE • Laparoscopic clip applier; for vessels and arteries through trocar

VARIETIES • 5 mm, 10 mm sizes; medium or large clip size

ALSO KNOWN AS • Endo clip

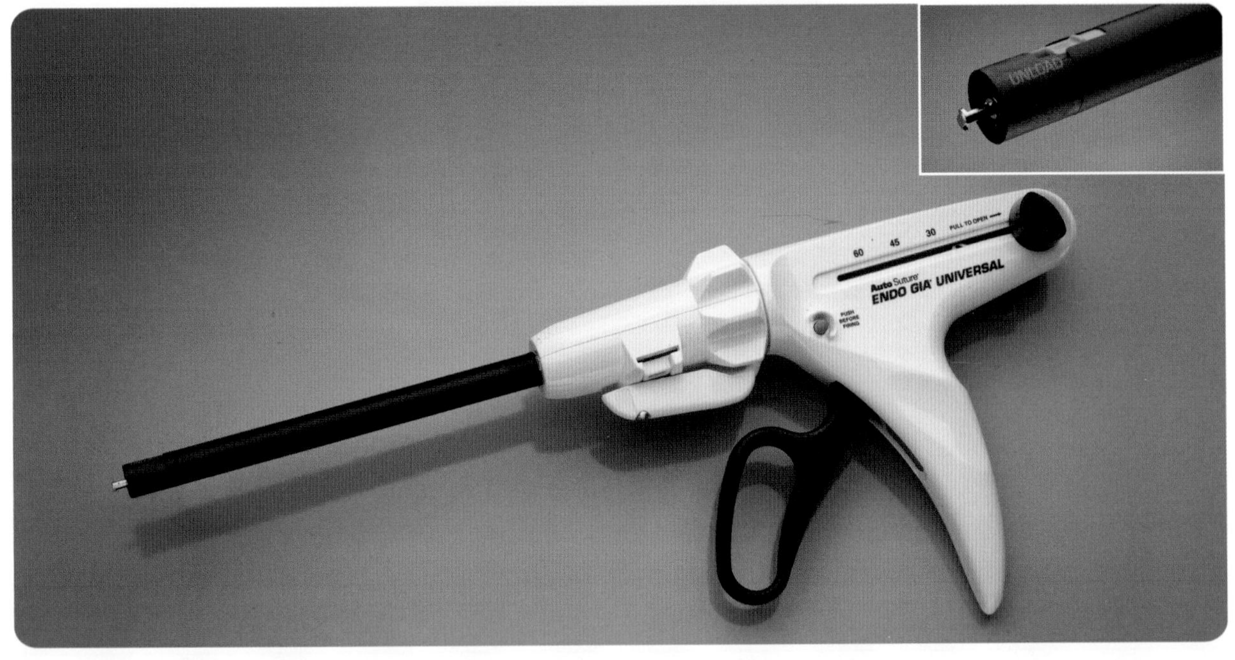
UNLOAD
60
45
30
PULL TO OPEN
Auto Suture
ENDO GIA UNIVERSAL
PUSH
BEFORE
FIRING

Linear Cutter/Endoscopic

USE • Laparoscopic stapler; to staple and cut tissue, arteries, veins, etc. through the trocar

VARIETIES • 30 mm, 45 mm, 60 mm sizes; reloads available in 2.5, 3.5, 4.8 sizes for tissue thickness; can be fired up to 8 times; disposable or reusable

ALSO KNOWN AS • Endo GIA, endo linear cutter

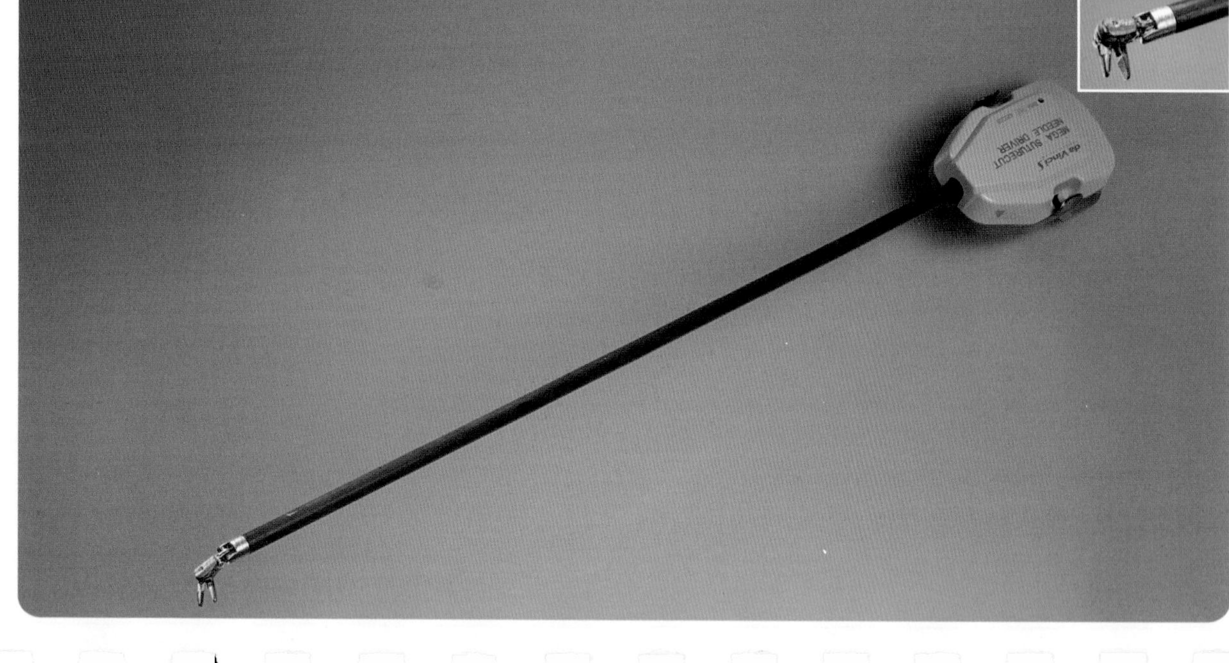
da Vinci S
MEGA SUTURECUT
NEEDLE DRIVER

Needleholder/Endowrist/Megasuture Cut Needle Driver/Robot

USE • To suture and to cut the suture during gynecology, general, urology, cardiovascular, and bariatric robotic-assisted minimally invasive surgery

VARIETIES • EndoWrist 5 mm instruments

ALSO KNOWN AS • EndoWrist instruments, miniaturized wristed instruments, patient EndoWrist instruments, robot needle holder

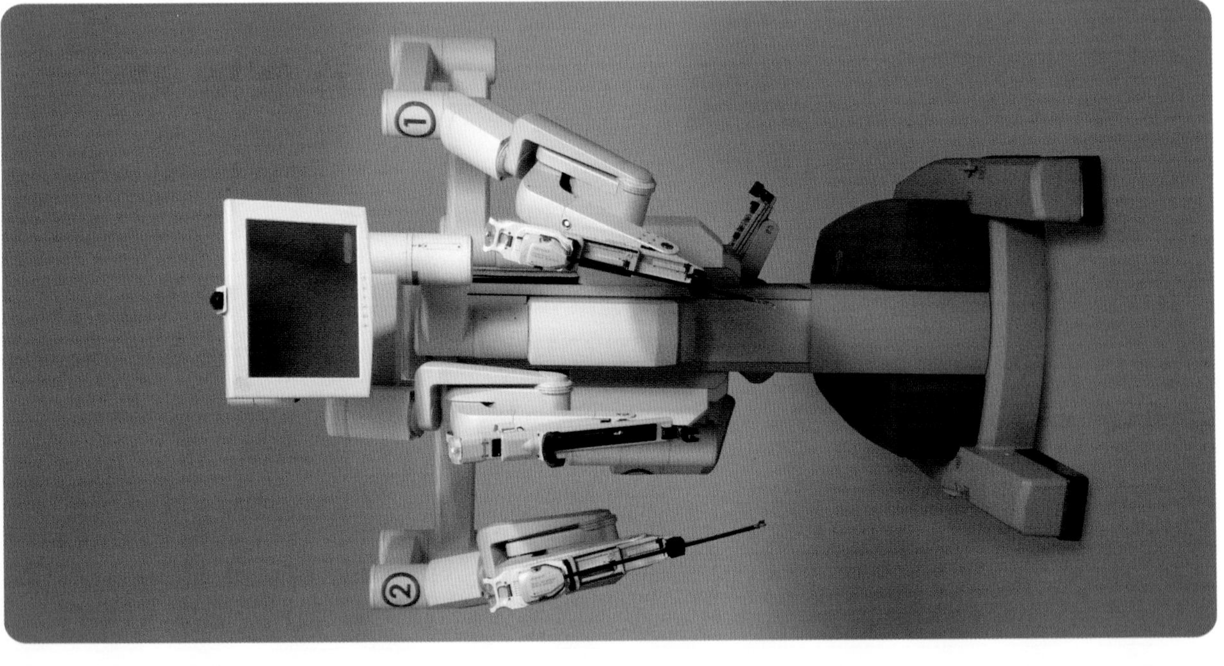
1
2

Patient Side Cart/Robot

USE
- To hold surgical wrist instruments during robotic-assisted minimally invasive surgery; every maneuver is directly controlled by the surgeon; system cannot be programmed or make decisions on its own; it consists of four arms, one of which can hold an endoscope/camera and the other two to three arms can hold the wrist instruments or move obstructions out of the way (acting as the surgeon's hands); the robotic arms are other tools used by the surgeon like a scalpel or clamp

VARIETIES
- Contains four interactive robotic arms

ALSO KNOWN AS
- da Vinci Surgical System, the robot: www.davincisurgery.com/davinci-surgical_system/features.html

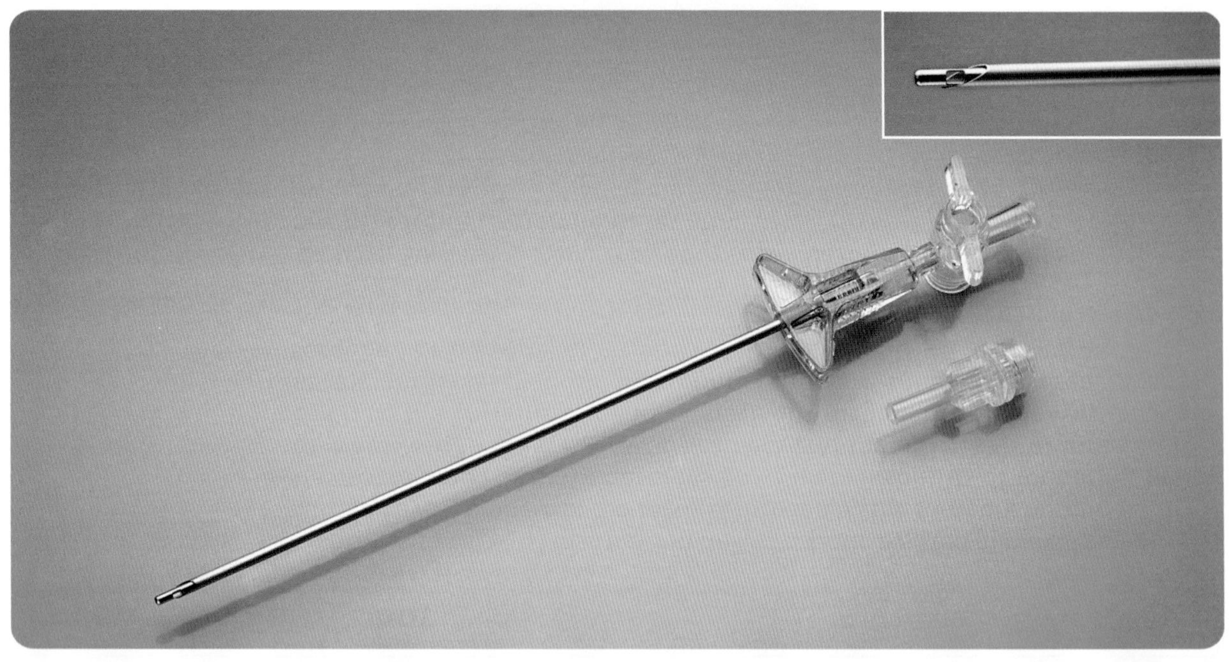

Pneumoperitoneum Needle

USE • To puncture and enter abdomen to insufflate and cause pneumoperitoneum; laparoscopy

VARIETIES • 120 mm, 150 mm sizes; single use instrument

ALSO KNOWN AS • Surgineedle, Veress needle

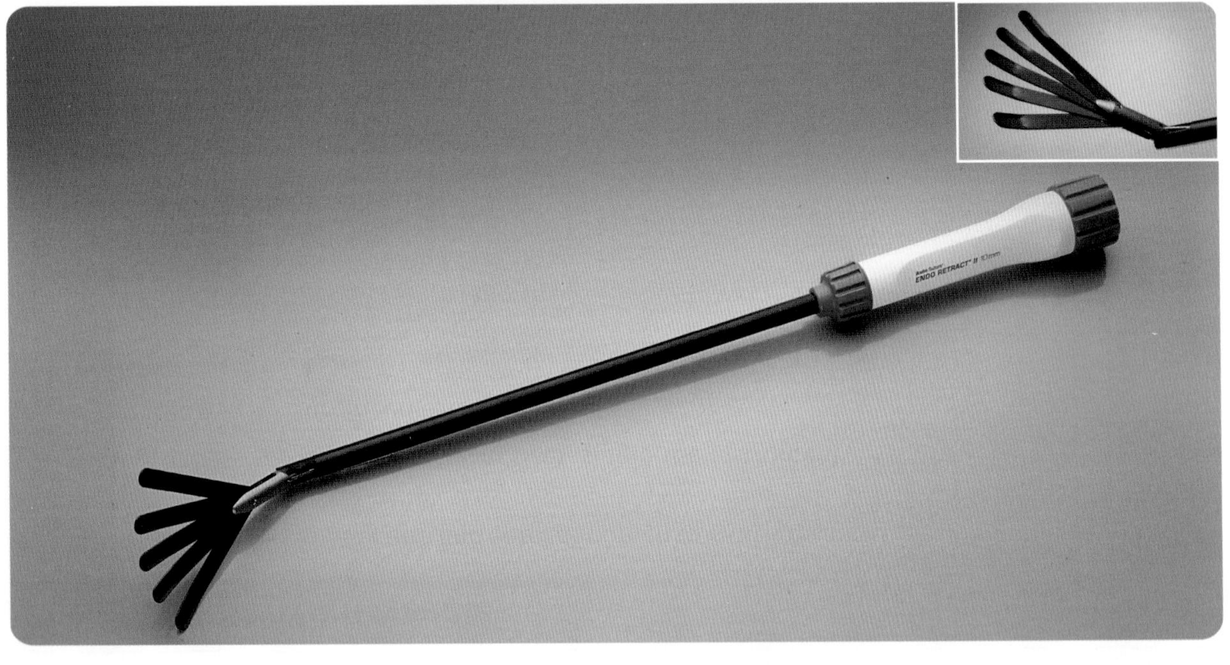
ENDO RETRACT* II 10mm

Retractor/Endoscopic

USE • Dissecting, cutting, retracting, and grasping various organs and vessels

VARIETIES • Endo retract, endo shears, endo grasp, endo fan, endo babcock, endo dissect, endo paddle; different lengths and single use

ALSO KNOWN AS • Hand instruments, laparoscopic hand instruments, laparoscopic retractors

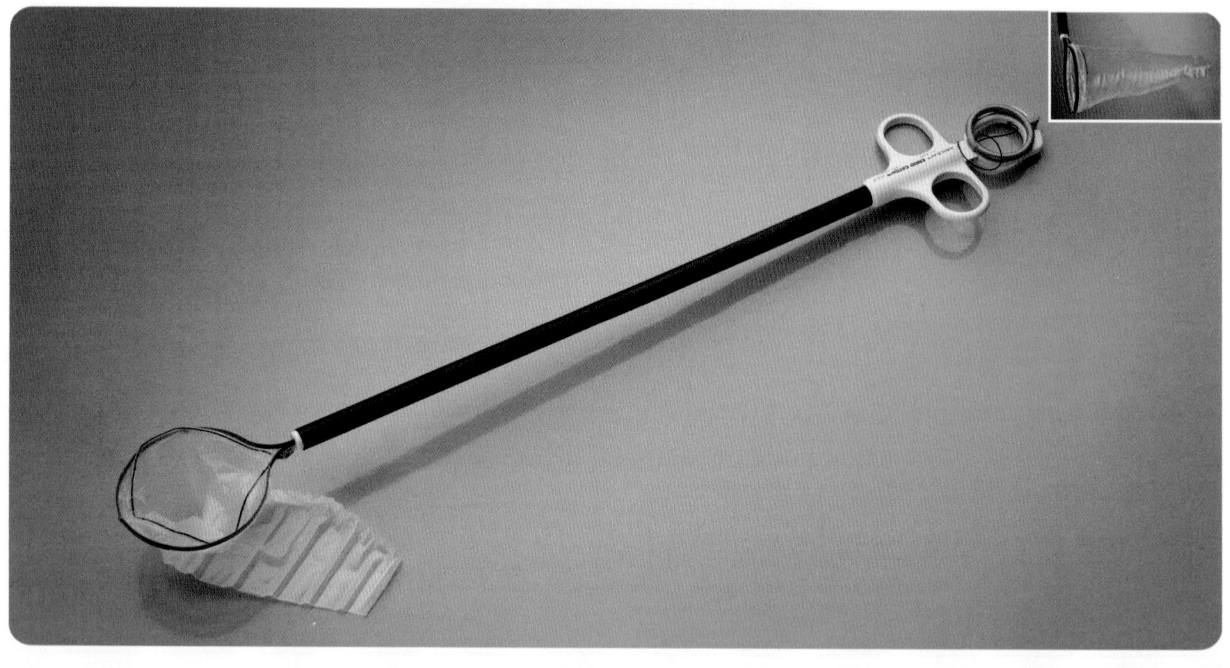
ENDO CATCH

Retrieval Device/Endoscopic

USE • Laparoscopic bag for specimen retrieval

VARIETIES • 10 mm, 15 mm size

ALSO KNOWN AS • Endo catch, specimen bag, specimen pouch

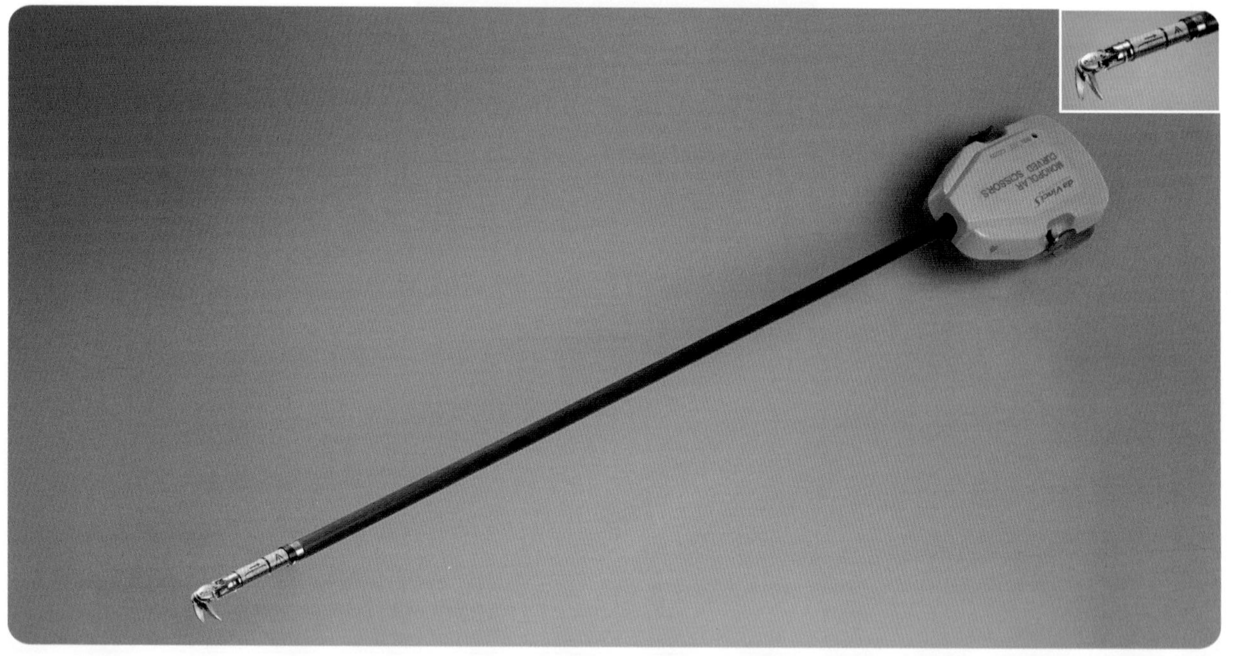
da Vinci S
MONOPOLAR
CURVED SCISSORS

Scissor/EndoWrist/Monopolar Curved Scissors/Robot

USE • To cut and dissect tissue during gynecology, general, urology, bariatric, and cardiovascular robotic-assisted minimally invasive surgery

VARIETIES • EndoWrist 5 mm instruments

ALSO KNOWN AS • EndoWrist instruments, miniaturized wristed instruments, patient EndoWrist instruments, robot scissor

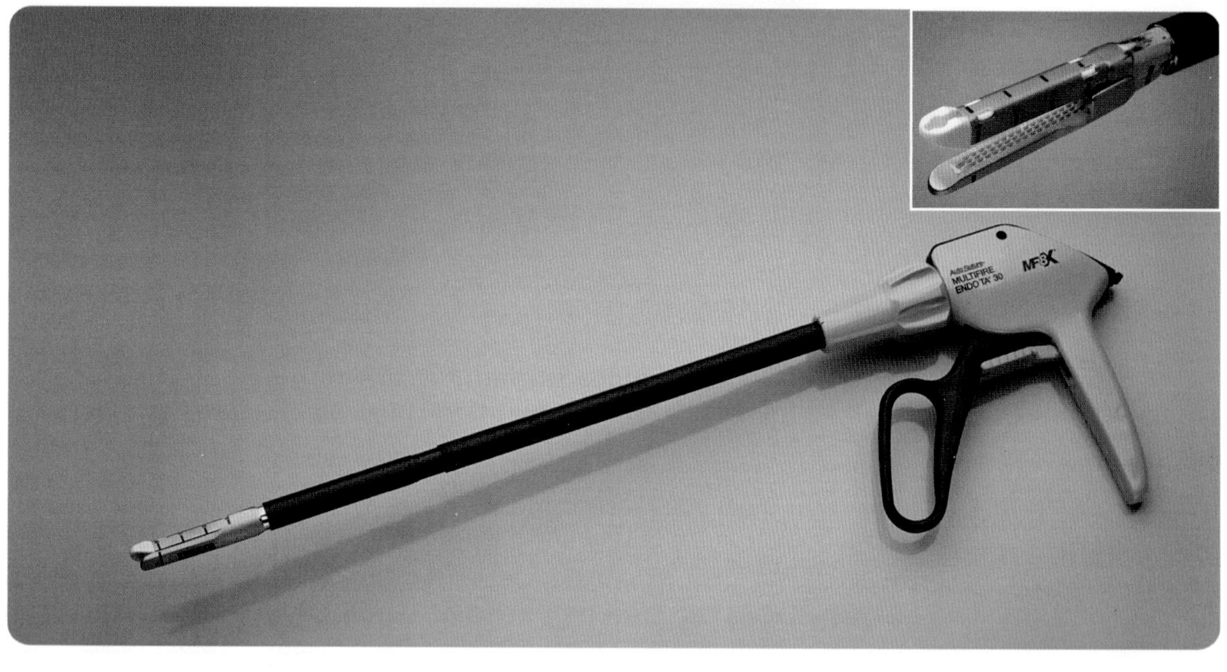
Auto Suture
MULTIFIRE
ENDO TA 30
MF8X

Stapler/Endoscopic/Multifire

USE • To staple tissue during endoscopic-assisted minimally invasive surgery

VARIETIES • Multifire staples; single use; 12 mm size; 2.5 and 3.5 length

ALSO KNOWN AS • Endo TA 30, Multifire Endo TA 30

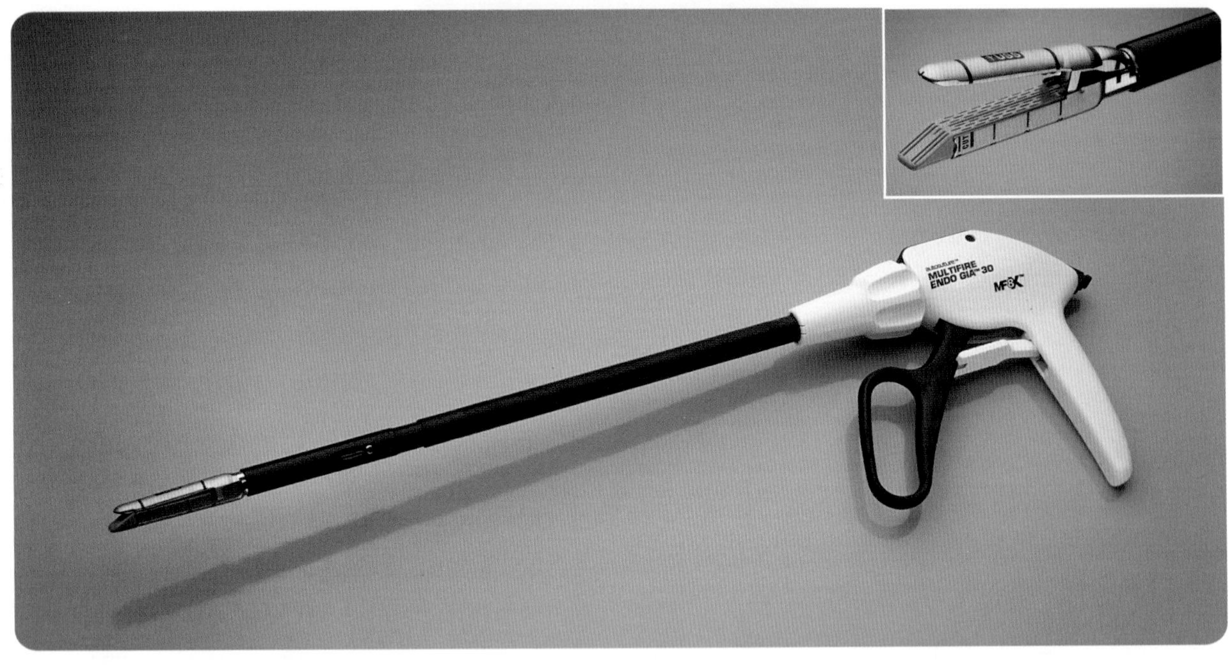
MULTIFIRE
ENDO GIA™ 30
CUT

Stapler/Endoscopic/Single Use

USE • Endoscopic stapler; application in abdominal, bariatric, gynecologic, pediatric, and thoracic surgery for resection, transection, and creation of anastomosis

VARIETIES • 30 mm, 45 mm, 60 mm sizes; 2.0, 2.5, 3.5, 4.8 loading units; can be fired up to 25 times

ALSO KNOWN AS • Endo GIA universal, single-use stapler

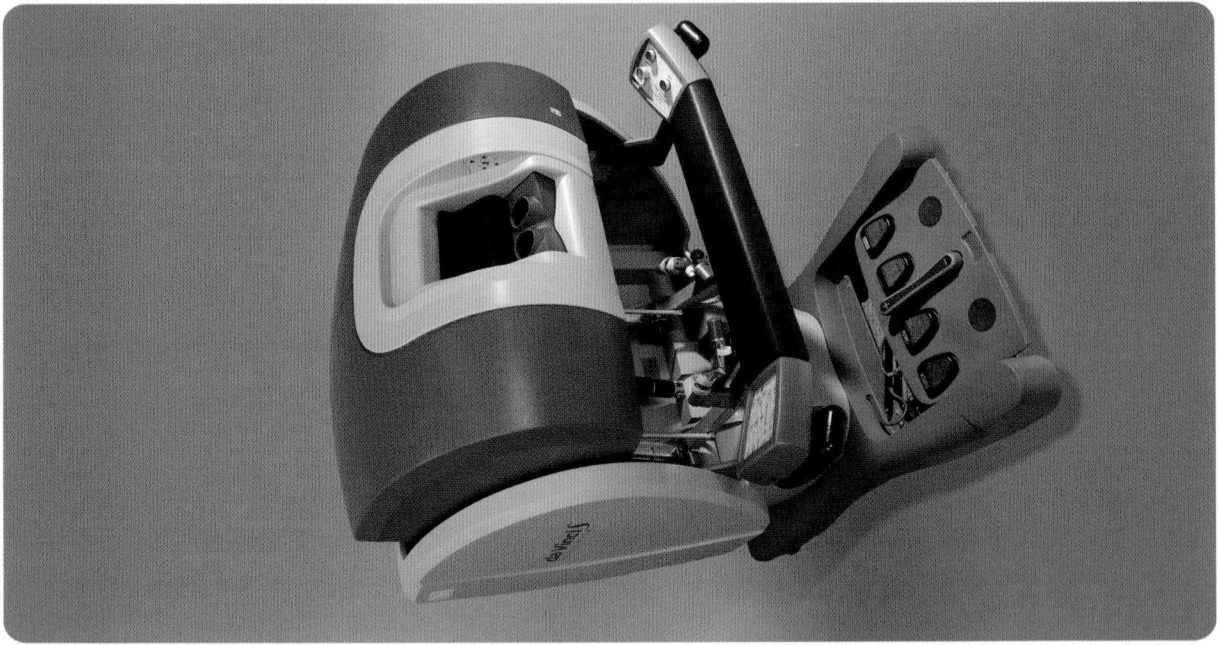

Surgeon Console/Robot

USE • Cardiovascular, gynecology, general, and urology robotic-assisted minimally invasive surgery; to enhance the surgeon's ability to perform delicate procedures through tiny surgical openings and suture with precision; minimally invasive option for complex surgical procedures; surgeon sits at the console away from the patient, looks through a viewfinder, and operates the master controls that work like forceps while viewing a highly magnified 3D image of the body's interior with bright, crisp images; the system translates the surgeons hands, wrist, and finger movements as surgical instruments inside the patient.

VARIETIES • One console

ALSO KNOWN AS • da Vinci Surgical System, the robot: www.davincisurgery.com/davinci-surgical_system/features.html

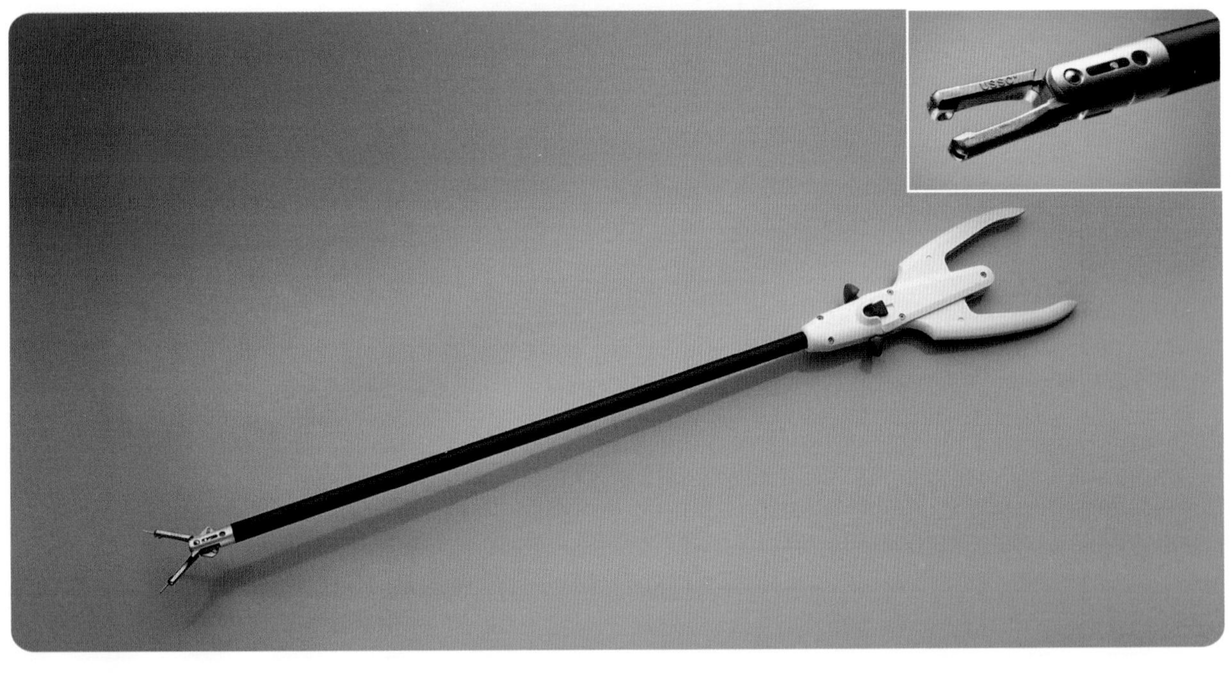
USSC

Suture Device/Endoscopic

USE • Laparoscopic suturing device; sutures defects, bleeders, approximates tissue; used for gastric bypass procedure

VARIETIES • Loaded with various suture materials, sizes, and different lengths

ALSO KNOWN AS • Endo stitch

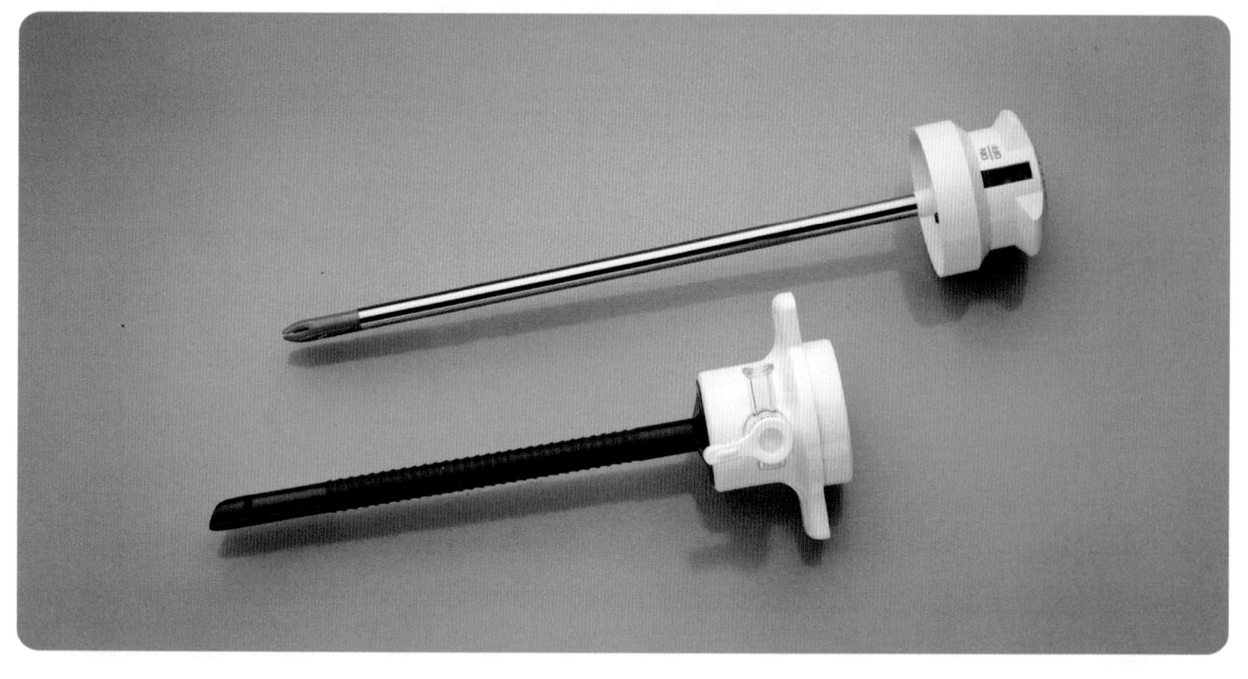
ON
OFF

Trocars/Bladeless/Cannula

USE • To puncture and enter the abdomen; as a sleeve for various instruments; laparoscopy

VARIETIES • 5, 8, 11, 12, 15 mm sizes; 70 mm, 100 mm, 150 mm lengths; fixation or smooth cannula included and universal seal

ALSO KNOWN AS • Sleeve, trocar, versaport

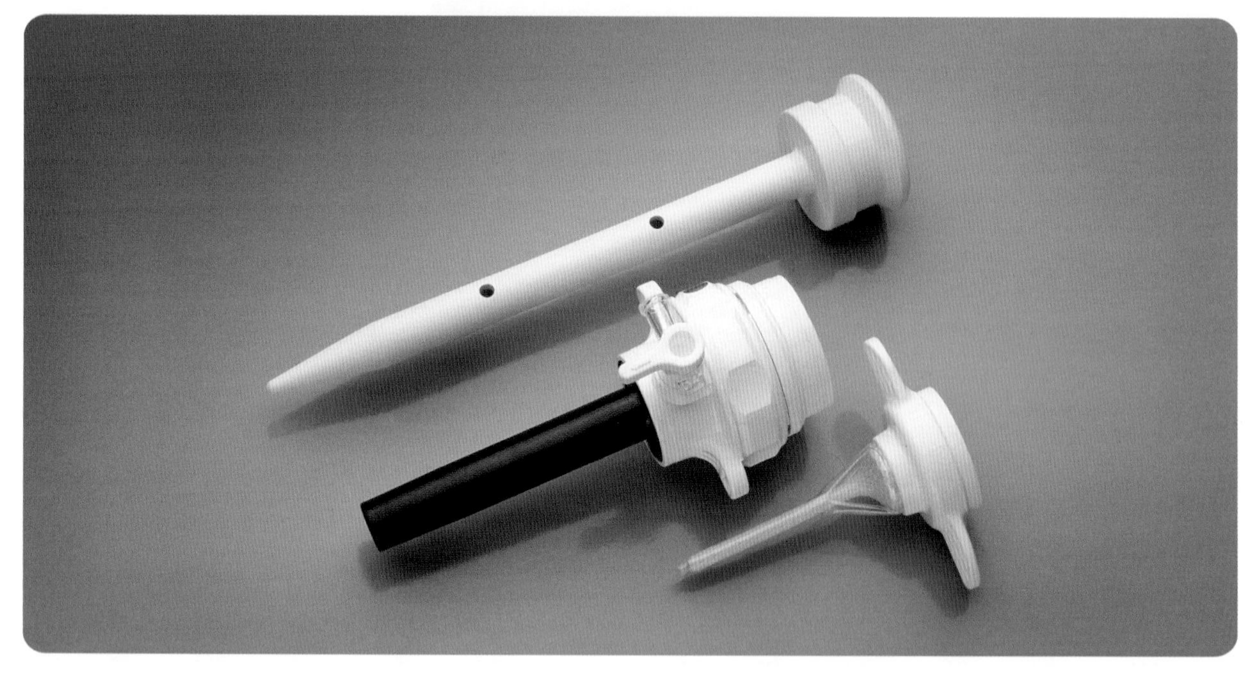

Trocars/Bladeless/Cannula/Dilator

USE • To access system for bladeless abdominal entry; laparoscopy

VARIETIES • 5, 11, 12, 15 mm sizes; 70 mm, 110 mm, and 150 mm lengths; cannula, dilator, and sleeve included

ALSO KNOWN AS • Bladeless trocar, cannula, and dilator set; VersaStep

CHAPTER 9

Internal Staplers

Internal staplers are used in place of sutures in open surgical procedures. They are more accurate, consistent, and much faster to use than suturing by hand. The staple line can be straight, curved, or circular, and can be used to connect or remove parts of the bowel or lung.

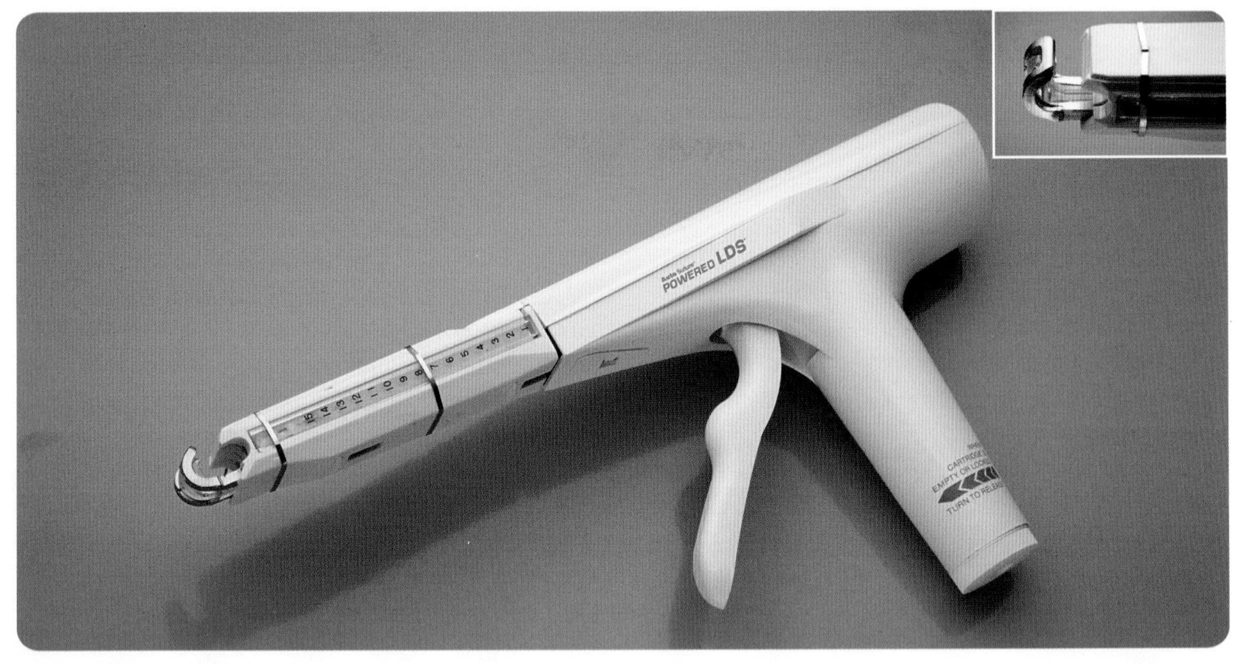
Auto Suture
POWERED LDS
TURN TO RELEASE

Clip Appliers/Large/Open Surgery

USE • To ligate and divide (cut) vessels, omentum, mesentery, fat

VARIETIES • One size; 15 clips; single use; reusable; powered

ALSO KNOWN AS • LDS, powered LDS

320

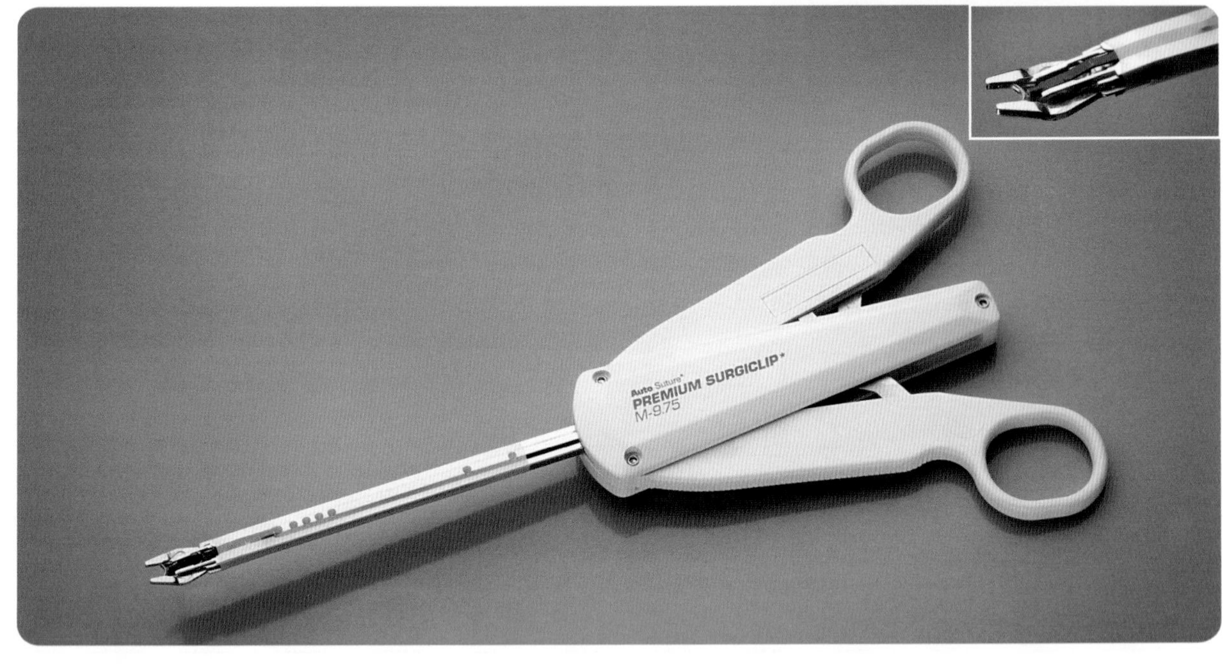

Clip Appliers/Small/Open Surgery

USE • To ligate and clip small arteries, veins, vessels

VARIETIES • Small, medium, large size; single use; automatic

ALSO KNOWN AS • Clip, premium surgiclip, surgiclip

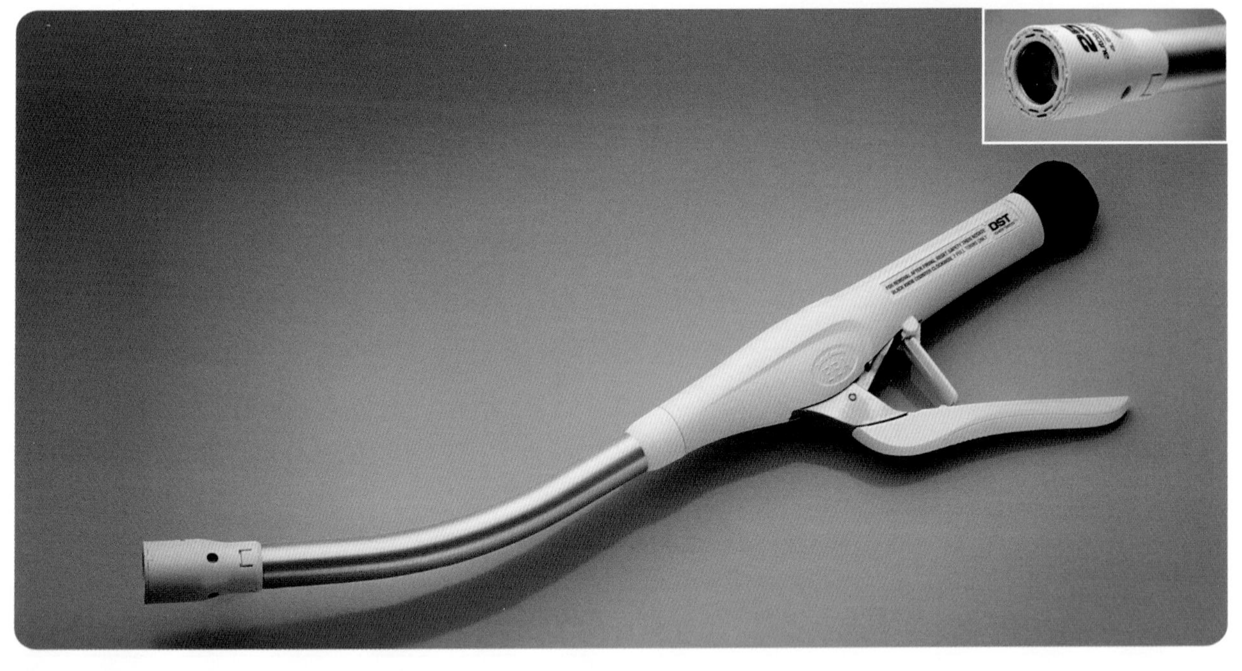
DST

Stapler/Open/Circular

USE • Circular anastomosis of rectum to bowel, esophagus to stomach; staples and cuts

VARIETIES • 21, 25, 28, 31, 34 mm sizes; no reloads; size of stapler depends on size of tissue; tilt top; single use

ALSO KNOWN AS • EEA

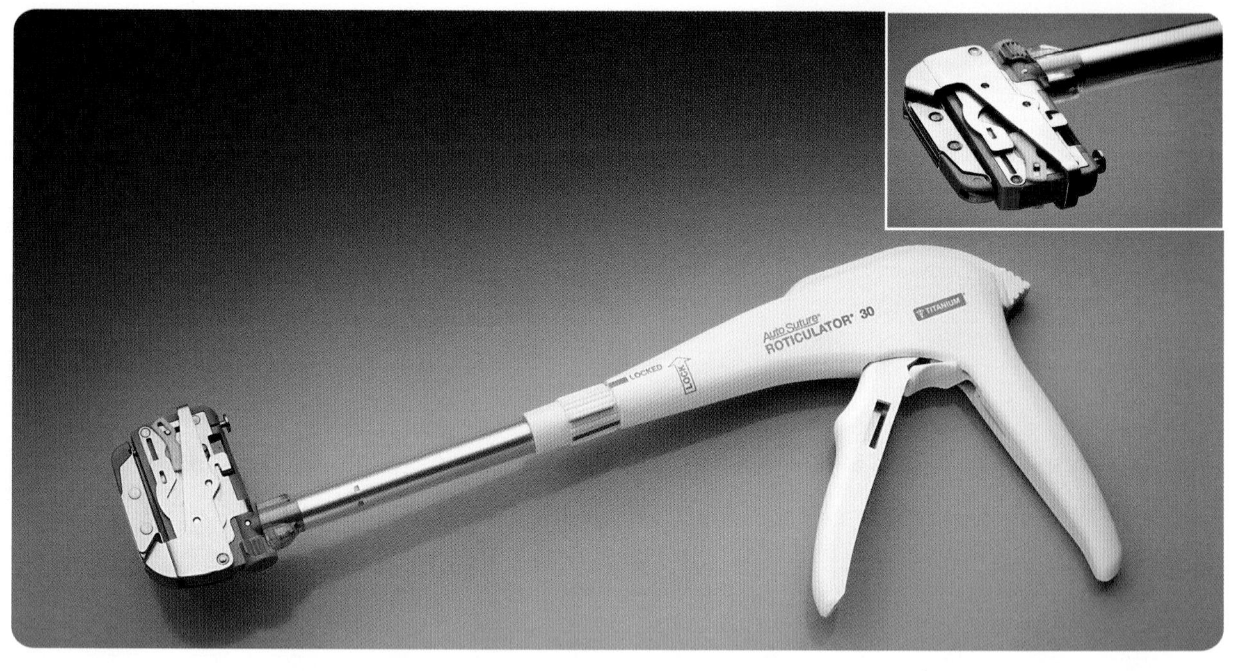
Auto Suture®
ROTICULATOR® 30
TITANIUM
LOCKED
LOCK

Stapler/Open/Rotatable

USE • Artery, vein, lung, stomach, colon resection; vascular and bariatric surgery

VARIETIES • 30, 45, 60, 90 mm sizes; reloads available in all sizes; TA roticulator 30, 55 (articulates and rotates); TA poly roticulator (articulates and rotates; absorbable staples); single use and reusable

ALSO KNOWN AS • TA, multifire TA

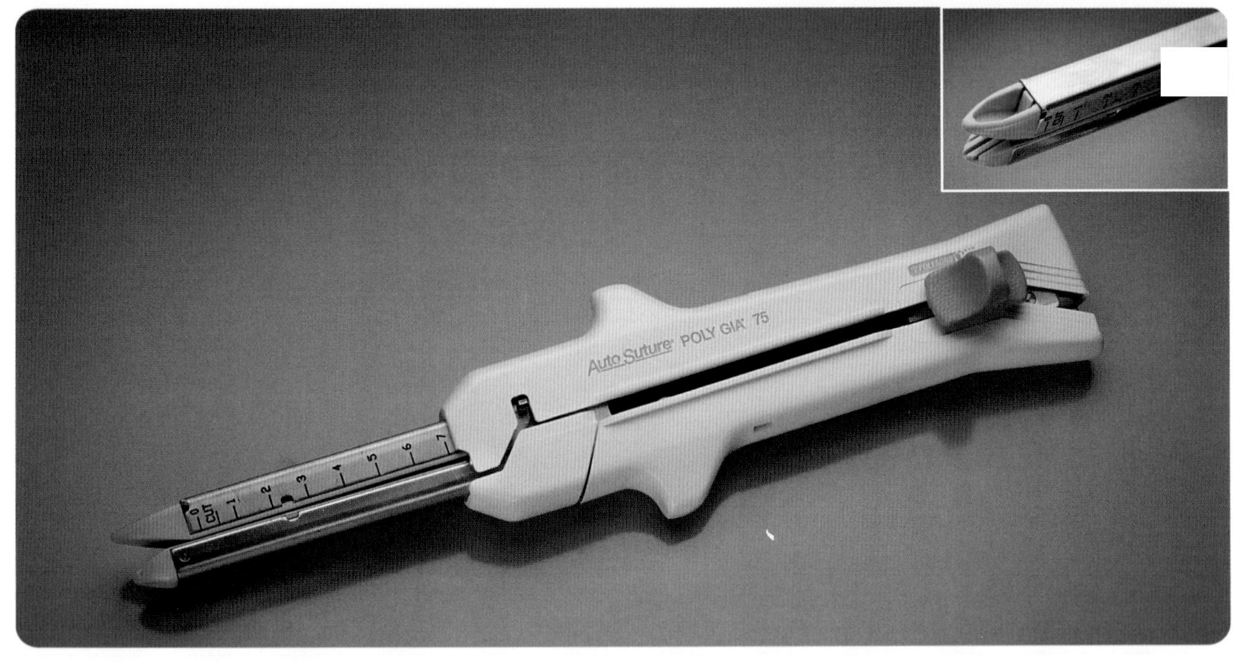
Auto Suture POLY GIA 75
0
CUT
1
2
3
4
5
6
7

Stapler/Open/Straight

USE • Gastrointestinal anastomosis, lung, stomach, colon resection; staples and cuts

VARIETIES • GIA 30, 60, 75, 80 mm sizes; reloads available in all sizes; SGIA (knifeless); poly GIA (absorbable staples); multifire; single use

ALSO KNOWN AS • GIA, poly GIA

CHAPTER 10 Surgical Power Tools

Surgical power tools are instruments specific to surgical procedures and many different surgical specialties. They are used mostly for small and large bone procedures. Their functions include drilling, shaving, reaming, cutting, tunneling, and fixation. Surgical power tools can also provide side-to-side and back-and-forth motions to create cuts or fixation. They are battery powered or nitrogen operated along with interchangeable accessories.

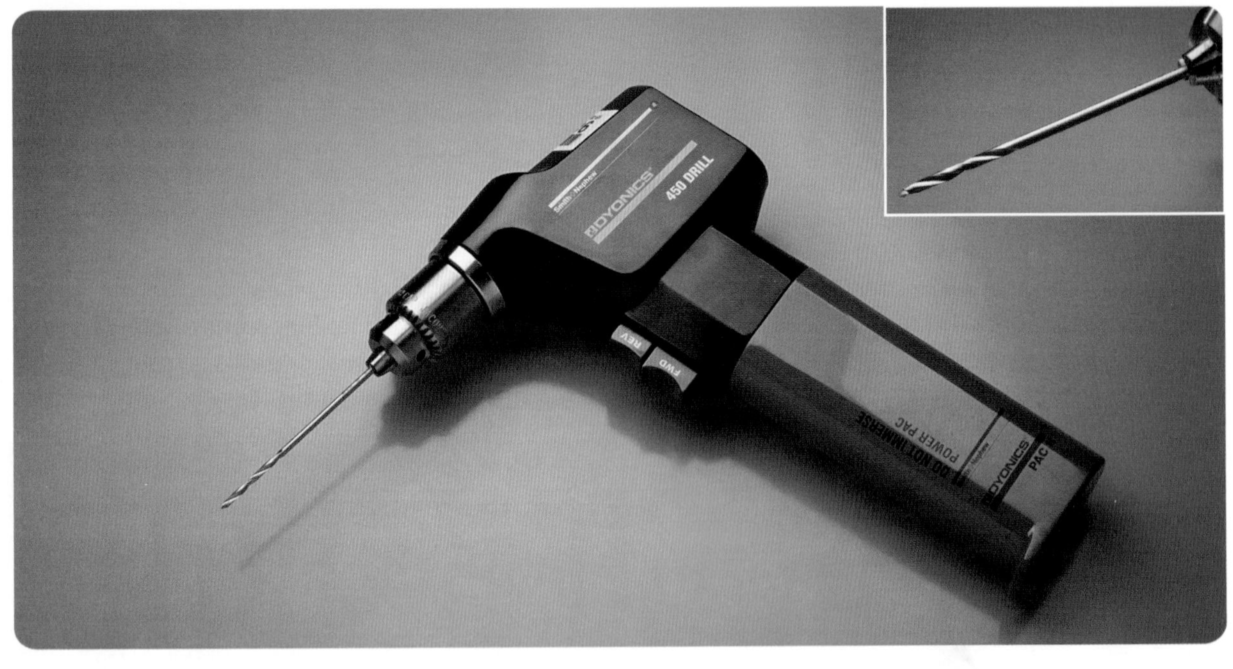

Smith & Nephew
DYONICS
450 DRILL
REV
FWD
DO NOT IMMERSE
POWER PAC
DYONICS
PAC

Drill/450

USE • To direct different size drill bits (2.0, 2.5, 3.2, etc.) into bone to receive an internal fixation screw that provides stabilization to the fracture site; to repair fractures of the upper extremity (hand and forearm) and fractures of the lower extremity (foot and ankle)

VARIETIES • Mostly battery operated; many manufacturers

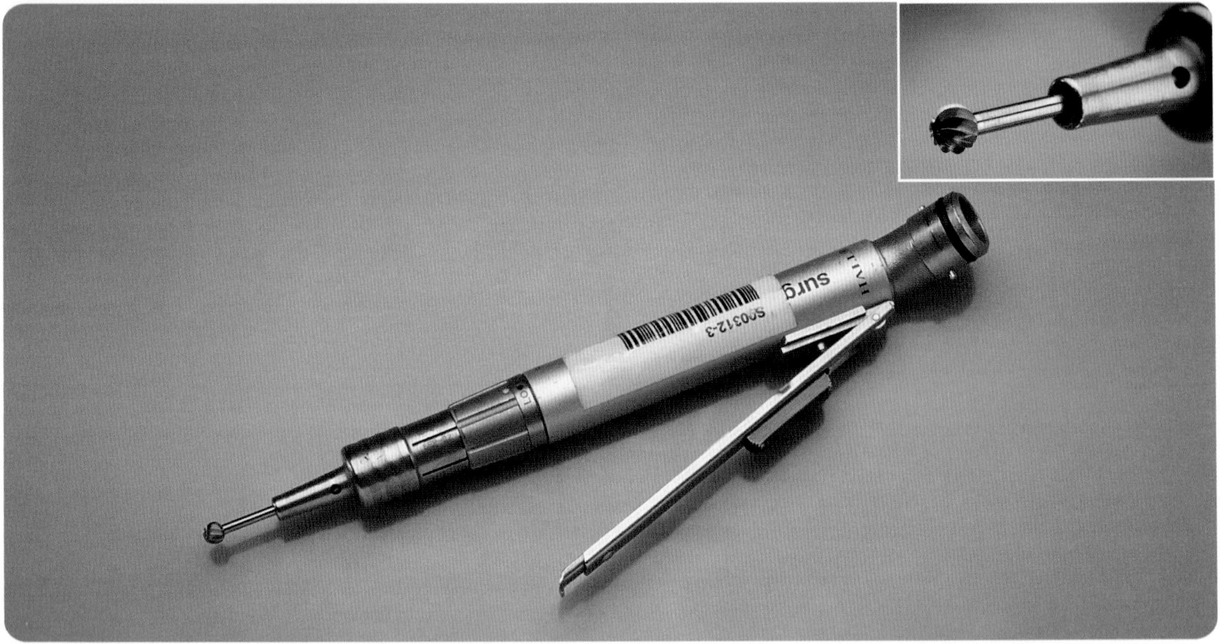

332

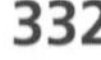

Drill/Surgairtome

USE • A high-speed drill that accepts different burrs to shave down bone; used in open shoulder surgery to shave down the acromium; also used in neurosurgery to contour types of allografts used in anterior cervical spinal fixation fusion cases; used in oral surgery to remove decayed bone in the mouth or mandible

VARIETIES • Mostly nitrogen powered; many manufacturers

ALSO KNOWN AS • High-speed burr drill

334

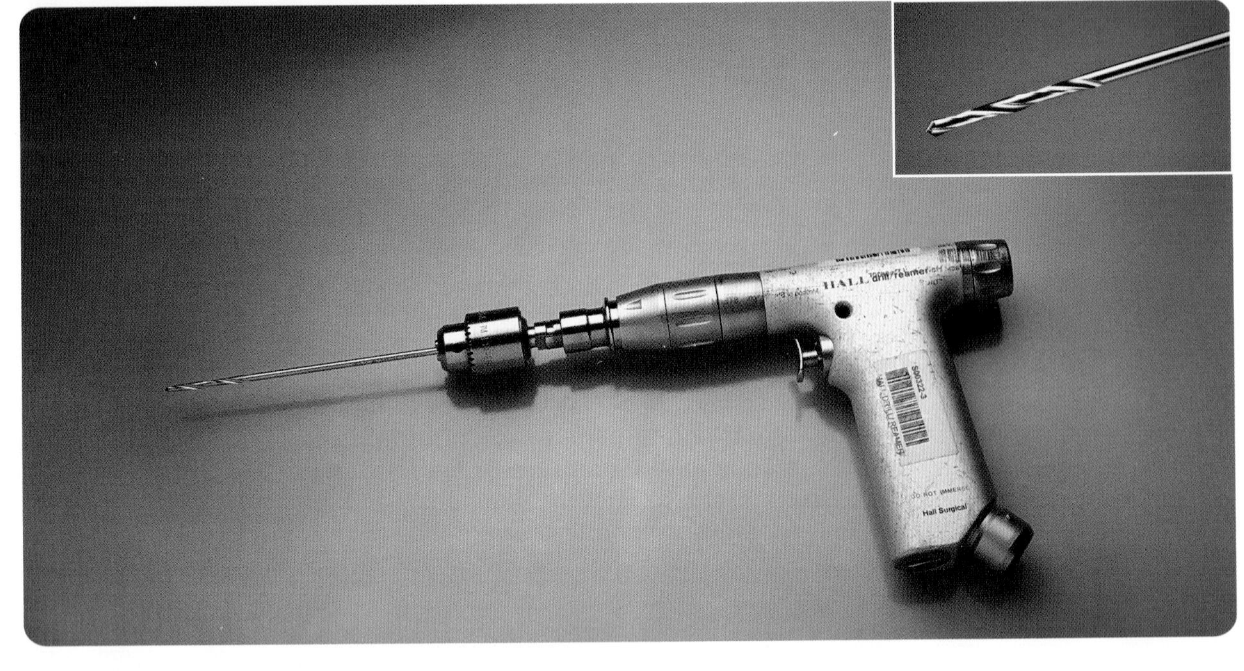

Driver/Reamer

USE • To direct different size drill bits into bone to prepare site for fixation screw that will provide stabilization to a fracture; used to ream the acetabulum and proximal femur during a total hip replacement; serves the same purpose during a total knee replacement by reaming the distal femoral and proximal tibial canals; used to prepare the femoral canal for an intramedullary rod/nail placement and can drill through the opening of the nail in the proximal and distal portions to lock the nail in place; used to drill the hole to sew in the rotator cuff during shoulder procedures

VARIETIES • Battery and nitrogen powered; many manufacturers

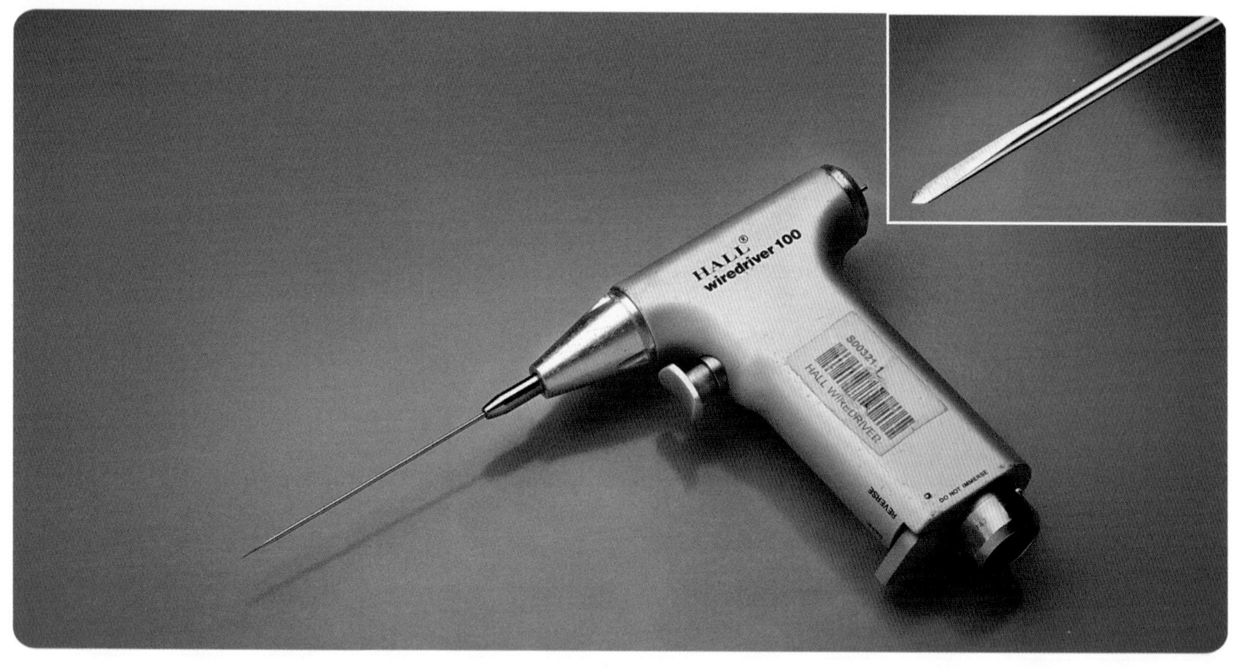
HALL®
wiredriver 100
S00321-L
HALL WIREDRIVER
REVERSE
DO NOT IMMERSE

Driver/Wire

USE • To guide various diameter K–wires (.062, .045, etc.) into bone to give temporary fixation; used during hand and sports medicine surgery and for lower extremity fractures (e.g., distal tibia/fibula and metatarsal/talus fractures)

VARIETIES • Battery and nitrogen powered; many manufacturers

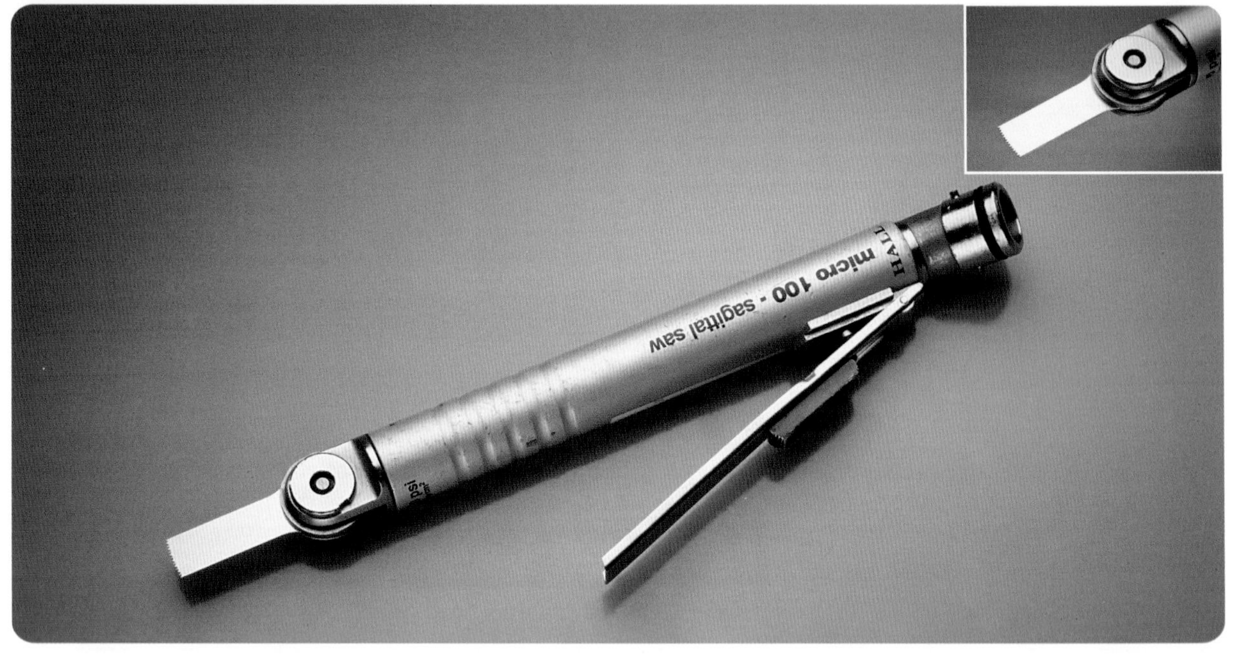
micro 100 - sagittal saw
psi

Saw/Microsagittal

USE • Provides a side-to-side motion to make cuts into or through small bone; used in orthopedics in upper extremity procedures (e.g., open reduction internal fixation (orif) of the shoulder, forearm, wrist, or hand); used on lower extremity procedures (e.g., distal tibia/fibula deformities or in sports medicine to trim down an allograft or foot surgery); used in neurosurgery to harvest iliac crest bone for anterior cervical spine fixation and fusion cases

VARIETIES • Mostly nitrogen powered; many manufacturers

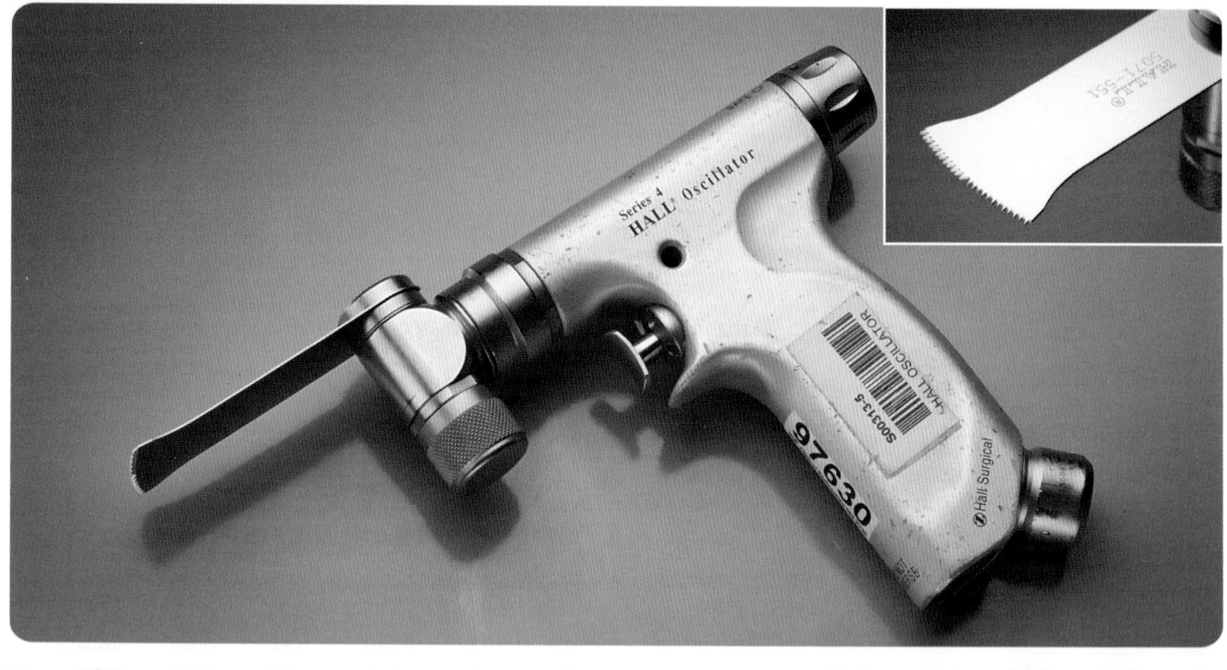
Series 4
HALL Oscillator
Hall Surgical
97630
S00313-5
HALL OSCILLATOR
HALL®
5071-551

Saw/Oscillating

USE • Provides a side-to-side motion to make an osteotomy or a cut into or through bone; used during total hip and total knee surgeries to remove diseased bone and to prepare the joint for the artificial prosthesis; used to correct a bone deformity or to perform an amputation (above or below the knee) secondary to trauma or osteomyelitis

VARIETIES • Battery and nitrogen powered; many manufacturers

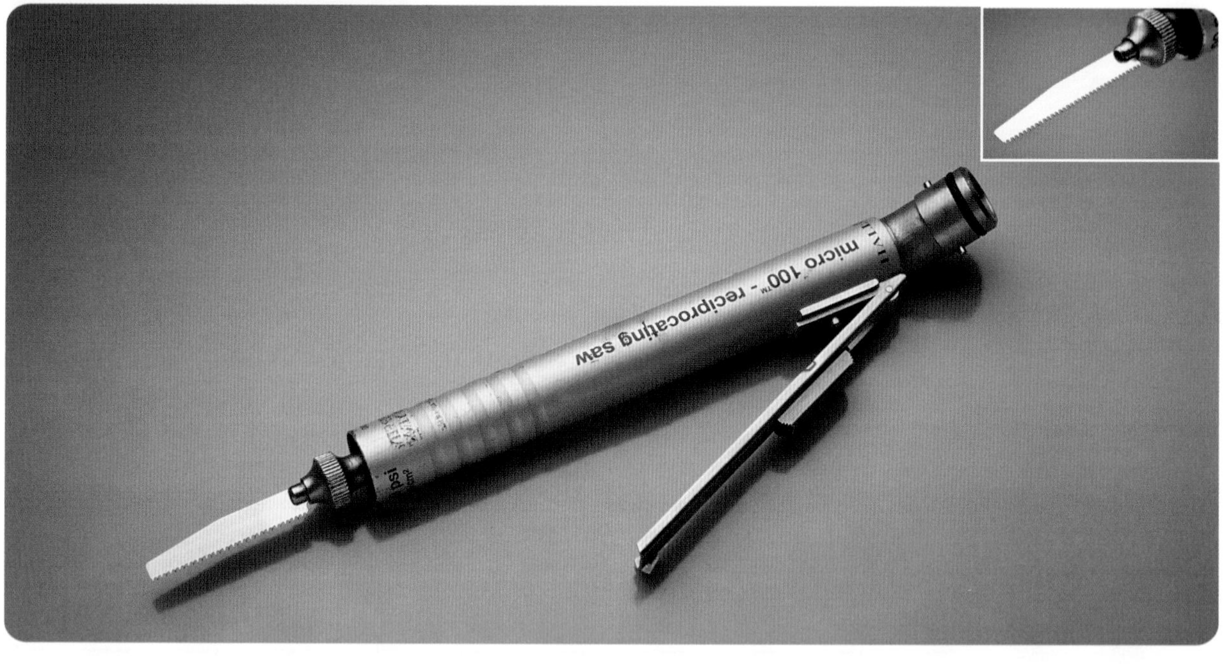
micro 100™ - reciprocating saw
psi

Saw/Reciprocating

USE • Provides a back-and-forth motion to make a cut through bone; in orthopedics, removes the femoral head in hip surgery to prepare the acetabulum for the prosthetic shell component; used for knee amputation procedures; cuts through the sternum to expose the heart in cardiac surgery

VARIETIES • Battery and nitrogen powered; many manufacturers

CHAPTER 11

Routine Instrument Sets

SET • Cardiac, CABG Tray, Robotic

USE • Mammary takedown

Instrument Index	Item(s)	PAR
Tray	Robot instrument tray	1
Forceps	Fine tissue	1
	Micro bipolar	1
Hook	Permanent cautery	1
Clip applier	Small	1

SET • Cardiac, Coronary

USE • CABG, pulmonary thromboendarterectomy, AVR, MVR, minimal invasive cardiac procedures

Instrument Index	Item(s)	PAR
Knife handles	Beaver, long	2
Scissors	60 degree coronary	1
	90 degree coronary	1
	125 degree coronary	1
	Jamison	1
Needle holders	Coronary	1
	Castro, round handle	1
	Castro, proximal	1
	Castro, distal	1
	Castro, distal nonlocker	1

Instrument Index	Item(s)	PAR
Forceps	Dietrichs	2
	Geralds	2
	7 ¼″ Mills	2
	8 ¼″ Mills	2
Miscellaneous	Fine right angle	1
	Parsonnet retractor	1
	Coronary probes, 1.0, 1.5, 2.0	3
	Webster cannula	1
	Sinker, pomeroy	1

SET • Cardiac, Mitral Valve Tray, Robotic

USE • Repair mitral leaflet

Instrument Index	Item(s)	PAR
Tray	Robot instrument tray	1
Scissors	Round tip scissors	1
Forceps	Fine tissue	1
	Resano	1
Hook	Valve	1
Retractor	Atrial	1
Needle driver	Large	1

SET • Cardiac, Open Heart

USE • CABG, AVR, MVR, sternal recurring pulmonary thromboendarterectomy, ventricular assist device implant

Instrument Index	Item(s)	PAR
Retractors	Favaloro-Morse	1
	Four-prong rakes	2
	Army-Navy	2
	Weitlaner	2
Miscellaneous	Clip appliers, small	3
	Clip appliers, medium	3
	Clip appliers, large	1
	Clip bar	1
	Rumel, regular	1
	Rumel, pediatric	1
	Aortic dialators, small, medium, large	3
	Frazier, 7 French, 10 French	2
	Nerve hook	1
	Ruler	1
	Grey pacer wires	2
	Ice cube tray	1

Continued

Cardiac, Open Heart—cont'd

Instrument Index	Item(s)	PAR
Scalpel handles	#3	2
	#7	2
Scissors	7″ Metzenbaum	2
	9″ Metzenbaum	2
	12″ Metzenbaum	1
	Long suture	1
	Straight Mayo	1
	Sternal wire cutter	1
	Nurse's	1
Forceps	Adsons	3
	Russians	3
	7″ DeBakey	4
	Blue burners	2

Instrument Index	Item(s)	PAR
Needle holders	Mayo-Hegar	4
	8″ Vascular	2
	10″ Vascular	2
	Serot	4
	Ravdin	2
	Sternal wire	2
	Tubing clamps	3
Clamps	Jackson	2
	Curved mosquitoes	4
	Straight mosquitoes	6
	Curved hemostats	10
	Straight hemostats	6
	Kellys	4

Kellys, long	2
Allises	8
Kochers	12
Criles	4
Mixtures	2
Sponge stick	2
Patent ductus	2
Crafoord	2
DeBakey clamp	2
Fogarty, extra large angled	1
Fogarty, large angled	1
Fogarty, small angle	1
Fogarty, small straight	1
Favalaro	1
Cooley, large	1
Derra	1
Cooley	1
Kay-Lambert	1
Towel clips, large	8
Towel clips, small	2
Beck	2

SET • General, Bariatric Tray, Robotic

USE • Robotic laparoscopic Nissen and gastric banding

Instrument Index	Item(s)	PAR
Tray	Robotic instrument	1
Needle driver	Suture cut	1
	Large	1
Grasper	Double fenestrated	1
Hook	Permanent cautery	1
Forcep	Cadiere	2

SET • General, Dissecting

USE • Breast biopsy, hernia repair, wide excision of lesions, amputations, hemorrhoidectomy

Instrument Index	Item(s)	PAR
Retractors	Sharp Senn	2
	Army-Navy	2
	Three-prong dull rakes	2
	Three-prong sharp rakes	2
	Deaver, shallow	2
	7½″ Weitlaner, blunt	1
	Bands	2
Forceps	5½″ Smooth dressing	2
	5½″ Tissue, 1 × 2 teeth	2
	Adson, tissue with 1 × 2 teeth	2

Instrument Index	Item(s)	PAR
Scissors	7″ Metzenbaum	1
	5¾″ Metzenbaum, baby	1
	6″ Mixter, suture	1
	6″ Nurse's, straight operating	1
Scalpel handles	#3	2
	#7	1
Clamps	5½″ Hemostat, curved	10
	5½″ Hemostat, straight	6
	5″ Mosquito, curved	6
	5″ Mosquito, straight	6

Continued

General, Dissecting—cont'd

Instrument Index	Item(s)	PAR
	6 ¼″ Kelly, Rochester-Péan	6
	6 ¼″ Kocher, Rochester-Ochsner	6
	6″ Allis, tissue forceps with 4 × 5 teeth	6
	9″ Sponge forcep	1
	5 ¼″ Backhaus towel clip	8
Needle holders	5″ Mayo-Hegar, plastic	2
	7″ Mayo-Hegar	2
Suction tips	8 French Frazier	1
Miscellaneous	8″ Probe with eye	1
	5 ½″ Groove director	1

SET • General, Laparotomy

USE • Small bowel obstruction, appendectomy, modified radical mastectomy, gastrectomy, hepatic lobectomy, pancreatic jejunostomy

Instrument Index	Item(s)	PAR
Retractors	Shallow	2
	Deep	2
	Broad	2
	Kelly Richardson 2½″ × 3″	1
	1½″ Wide malleable	1
	Band	3
Forceps	10″ Smooth dressing	2
	5½″ Smooth dressing	2
	5½″ Tissue with 1 × 2 teeth	2
	Adson, tissue with 1 × 2 teeth	2
	8″ Russian, tissue	2
	9½″ DeBakey, vascular tissue	2
Scissors	7″ Metzenbaum	2
	8″ Metzenbaum, long	1
	6″ Nurse's, straight operating	1

Continued

General, Laparotomy—cont'd

Instrument Index	Item(s)	PAR
	6 ¼″ Mixter, suture	1
	8″ Sims, long suture	1
Scalpel handles	#3	2
	#7	1
	#3, long	1
Suction tips	Andrew pincher	1
	10 French Frazier	1
Needle holders	5″ Mayo-Hegar, plastic	2
	7″ Serot	2
	8″ Mayo-Hegar, gold handle	4
Clamps	5 ½″ Hemostat, curved	10
	5 ½″ Hemostat, straight	8
	6 ¼″ Kelly (Rochester-Péan)	6
	6 ¼″ Kocher (Rochester-Ochsner)	10
	6″ Allis, tissue forcep	5
	6 ¼″ Babcock	4
	7 ¼″ Schnidt (Crile)	4
	7 ¼″ Adson, curved (fine Crile)	2

	9″ Mixter	4	Miscellaneous	8″ Probe with eye	1
	9″ Mixter, fine (Gemini)	2		5½″ Groove director	1
	9″ Kelly, long (Péan)	6		10½″ Valve hook, gastric	1
	9½″ Babcock, long	4		Clip applier, large	2
	10″ Allis, long with 5 × 5 teeth	4		Clip applier, medium	2
	9″ Sponge forcep	2		Clip bar	1
	5¼″ Backhaus towel clip	3			

SET • General, Major, Endoscopic

USE • Laparoscopic hernia, laparoscopic cholecystectomy, laparoscopic appendectomy, laparoscopic Nissen fundoplication

Instrument Index	Item(s)	PAR
Graspers	Allis rachet	2
Forceps	Large grasping	1
	Dissecting	1
Dissectors	Maryland 10 mm	1
	5 mm	1
Clamps	Dorsey bowel 1 mm	1
	Endo loop passer	1
Rod	Pleatman sac	1
Cleaner	Brush	1
Retractors	Army-Navy	2
	"S"	2

Instrument Index	Item(s)	PAR
Cups	Aluminum	2
Cord	Monopolar	1
Adapter	Male	1
Tubing	CO_2	1
Probes	Nezhat irrigation probe	1
Miscellaneous	Scope warmer	1
	Scope warmer base	1
	Black warmer cap	1
	Video equipment	
	Light cord	1
	0 degree scope	1

SET • General, Plastics

USE • Facelift, rhinoplasty, blepharoplasty, brow lift, breast augmentation

Instrument Index	Item(s)	PAR
Retractors	Skin hooks	2
	Senn	2
Scissors	Doctor's, short	1
	Nurse's	1
	Iris	1
	Brown	1
Forceps	Adson-Brown	1
	Adson	2
	Brown	1
	Smooth	1
Clamps	Mosquitoes, curved	10
	Mosquitoes, straight	8
	Hemostats, straight	2
	Kochers	2
	Allises	6
	Towel clips, small	6
	Towel clips, large	4
Needle holders	Brown	2
	Webster	2
Knife handle	#3	2
Suction tips	Plastic	1
	Frazier	1
Miscellaneous	Ruler	1
	Cups	3

SET • General, Plastics, Endoscopic

USE • Brow lift, facelift

Instrument Index	Item	PAR
Retractors	Periosteal spreader	1
	Nerve retractor, left	1
	Nerve retractor, right	1
Scissors	Endoscopic forehead, curved	1
Forceps	Endoscopic, left	1
Dissectors	Temporalis	1
	Marginalis	1
	Periosteal elevator	1
Miscellaneous	Endoscopic cannula, 5 mm	1
	Light cord, 5 mm	1
Video	30 degree scope, 5 mm	1

SET • General, Radical Mastectomy

USE • Modified radical mastectomy; free flap muscle graft

Instrument Index	Item(s)	PAR
Retractors	Deaver, shallow	2
	Band	3
	Four-prong rakes, dull	2
	Thyroid rakes, dull	2
	Richardson, medium	1
	Richardson, large	1
	Vein	2
Forceps	Tooth	2
	Smooth	2
	Adson, toothed	2
	7″ Dental	2
	7″ Vascular	2
Scissors	Metzenbaum	2
	Nurse's	1
	Suture	1
	Doctor's, large	1
Needle holders	Gold handle	4
	Plastic	2

Continued

General, Radical Mastectomy—cont'd

Instrument Index	Item(s)	PAR
Clamps	Hemostat, curved	15
	Hemostat, straight	10
	Kellys	6
	Kochers	15
	Allises	4
	Mixtures	2
	Criles	6
	Towel clips	20

Instrument Index	Item(s)	PAR
Miscellaneous	#3 Knife handle	3
	Sponge stick	1
	Hemoclip, large	2
	Hemoclip, medium	2
	Clip bar	1

SET • Gynecology, D & C Tray

USE • D & C, vaginal biopsies, cone biopsies, cerclage, D & E

Instrument Index	Item(s)	PAR
Deaver	Narrow	2
Speculums	Duckbill	1
	Weighted	
Miscellaneous	Metal catheter	1
	7″ Needle holder	1
	Mayo scissors	1
	#3 Knife handle	1
	Hemostats, straight	4
	Allises, long	2
	Double-toothed tenaculum	2
	Polyp forceps, small	1
	Hegar dilator, small	1
	Tooth forcep, medium	1
	Smooth forcep, medium	1
	Curette, Tieman	1
	Curette, small	1
	Curette, medium	1
	Curette, large	1
	Sims, small	1
	Sims, large	1

Continued

Gynecology, D & C Tray—cont'd

Instrument Index	Item(s)	PAR
	Sims, handled	1
	Sponge sticks	2
	Sound	1
	Spoon	1
	Gauzed metal basin	1
	Metal cup	1
	Metal pitchers	2
	Wylie tenaculum	1

SET • Gynecology, Endoscopic

USE • Laparoscopic oophorectomy, laparoscopic vaginal hysterectomy, tubal ligation, laparoscopic removal of ectopic pregnancy

Instrument Index	Items	PAR
Retractors	Army-Navy	2
	"S"	2
Miscellaneous	Scope warmer	1
	Scope warmer base	1
	5 mm wand	1
Video	Allis ratchet graspers, 5 mm	1
	Maryland dissectors, 5 mm	1
	Dorsey bowel clamp, 5 mm	1
	Nezhat Dorsey dissection grasper, 3 mm	1
	Nezhat Dorsey irrigation aspirator, 5 mm sleeve	1
	Kleppinger bipolar forcep	1
	Bipolar cord	2
	Laser stripper .025	1

Continued

Gynecology, Endoscopic—cont'd

Instrument Index	Items	PAR
	Laser fiber insert 33 cm	1
	Laser fiber cleaver	1
	Ovarian grasper	1
	0 degree scope, 10 mm	1
	Light cord	1

SET • Gynecology, Gyn Tray, Robotic

USE • Robotic laparoscopic-assisted hysterectomy, myomectomy, supracervical abdominal hysterectomy, blind uterus resection, tubal anastomosis, resection uterine horn, bilateral salpingo oophorectomy

Instrument Index	Item(s)	PAR
Tray	Robotic instrument	1
Forceps	Dissecting	1
	Cadiere	1
	Fenestrated bipolar	1
Needle driver	Large	1
	Suture cut	1
Scissors	Monopolar, curved	1

SET • Gynecology, Infertility

USE • Tubal reanastomosis, lysis of adhesions, tubal patency, ovarian cyst removal

Instrument Index	Item(s)	PAR
Retractors	O'Connor-O'Sullivan	1
	Retractor blades	3
	Wing nuts	2
	Kelly Richardson, small	2
	Kelly Richardson, medium	1
	Kelly Richardson, large	1
	Malleable	1
	Shoehorn	1
	Deaver, broad	2
	Deaver, narrow	2
	Bands	2
	Vein retractors	2

Instrument Index	Item(s)	PAR
Scissors	Mayo	1
	Metzenbaum, regular	1
	Strully	1
	Lincoln	1
	Vaginal dissecting	1
Suctions	Tonsil	1
	Abdominal	2
	Poole	1
	Frazier	1
Needle holders	8″ Mayo-Hegar	3
	Vascular diamond jaw	6
	Coronary	2

	7″ Serot	2
	Clip appliers, medium	1
	#3 Knife handles	2
	#3 Knife handle, large	1
	Skin hooks	2
	Cannulae	2
	Probes	2
	Freer elevator	1
Forceps	8″ Smooth	2
	8″ Tooth	2
	Adson, toothed	2
	7″ Diamond jaw	3
	10″ Diamond jaw	3
	7″ Potts, toothed tissue	2
	7″ Potts, smooth tissue	1

Clamps	Mosquitoes, curved	6
	Mosquitoes, straight	4
	Hemostats, curved	15
	Hemostats, straight	4
	Towel clips	6
	Kochers, straight	6
	8″ Allises	6
	Allises, short	4
	Kellys, long	6
	Williams	4
	Williams, long	4
	Mixters	4
	Criles	4
	Buxton	1
	Zeigler-Helman	1
	Sponge stick	1

SET • Gynecology, Laparoscopy

USE • Rule out ectopic pregnancy, lysis of adhesions, ovarian cyst, D & C, D & E

Instrument Index	Item(s)	PAR
Forceps	Kellys, long	1
	Short tooth	1
	Medium smooth	1
	Medium tooth	1
	Towel clips	3
	Allises, short	6
	Hemostats, straight	4
	Polyp, small	1
	Sponge sticks	2
Clamps	Tenaculum, long single tooth	1
	Tenaculum, short double tooth	2
	Hulka tenaculum	1
	Wiley tenaculum	1
Miscellaneous	Godell dilator	1
	Weighted speculum	1
	Metal catheter	1
	Sound	1
	Curette, large	1
	Curette, medium	1
	Curette, Tieman	1

Long metal pan	1
#3 Knife handle	1
Suture scissors, small	1
Needle holder, short	1
Sparkman cannula	1
Jarcho cannula	1
Acorn, small	1
Acorn, large	1
Triangle	1
Adson forcep	1
8 mm sheath and trocar	1
3 mm sheath and trocar	1
Metal pitcher	2
Metal cups	2
Washer	1
Rubber gas hose with adaptor	1
Handled Sims	1
Sims, large	1
Sims, medium	1

SET • Gynecology, Major

USE • Exploratory laparotomy, total abdominal hysterectomy, node sampling, pelvic adhesions, pelvic exenteration, ovarian cancer, omentectomy

Instrument Index	Item(s)	PAR
Scissors	8″ Metzenbaum, long	1
	8″ Sims, long suture	1
	6″ Nurse's, straight	1
	Preucel or Satinsky	1
Scalpel handles	#3, short	3
	#3, long	1
Needle holders	8″ Mayo-Hegar, gold handle	4
	10″ Mayo-Hegar	2
	6″ Mayo-Hegar	1
Clamps	5½″ Hemostat, curved	10
	5½″ Hemostat, straight	6

Instrument Index	Item(s)	PAR
	6″ Allis tissue forceps	4
	6¼″ Babcock, short	4
	9″ Kelly, long (Péan)	6
	7½″ Criles, Schnidt	4
	9″ Mixter	4
	9½″ Babcock, long	2
Retractors	Deaver, broad	2
	Deaver, narrow (deep)	2
	Malleable 1½″ wide ribbon	1
	Kelly Richardson 1½″ × 3″	1

	Kelly Richardson 2″ × 2½″	1
	Band	2
	O'Connor-O'Sullivan	1
	Retractor blades	3
	Retractor wing nuts	2
Forceps	12″ Smooth dressing	2
	12″ Tooth	2
	8″ Smooth dressing	2
	8″ Tooth	2
	Adson, toothed tissue (1 × 2)	2
Scissors	9″ Vaginal, long curved	1
	6¾″ Mayo, curved	1
	7″ Metzenbaum, regular	1
Clamps	Backhaus towel clips	6
	8¼″ Heaney, curved	4
	8½″ Heaney, straight	4
	Double tenaculums	6
	7¼″ Allises	6
	8″ Kochers	6
	8″ Uterine grasper, medium	1
	4″ Sponge forceps	3

SET • Gynecology, Vaginal

USE • Vaginal hysterectomy, vaginal and rectal prolapse

Instrument Index	Item(s)	PAR
Retractors	Weighted speculum, long	1
	Weighted speculum, short	1
	Sims, handled speculum	1
	Sims, large speculum	1
	Sims, medium speculum	1
	Deaver, narrow	2
	Heaney, right angle	2
	Bands	2
Needle holders	8″ Mayo-Hegar	2
	Heaney	2
Scissors	Nurse's, straight	1
	Metzenbaum, regular	1
	Vaginal dissecting	1
	Mayo	2
Forceps	8″ Tooth	2
	8″ Smooth	2

	Smooth, short	1		Mixters	2
	Adson, toothed	1		Tenaculums, Jacob	2
Clamps	Hemostats, curved	10		Tenaculum, single tooth	1
	Hemostats, straight	6		Kochers, curved	2
	Kellys, long	4		Babcocks, short	2
	8″ Allises	8		Babcocks, long	2
	Allises, short	6		Uterine grasper, medium	1
	Towel clips	6	Scalpel handles	#3 Knife handle, short	2
	Sponge sticks			#3 Knife handle, long	1
	Tenaculums, double tooth	4	Accessories	Metal pitchers	2
	Heaney, curved	6		Metal catheter	1
	9″ Zeppelin, extremely curved	2		Curette, Tiemans	1
	9″ Zeppelin, slightly curved	2		Uterine sound	1
	Zeppelin, straight	2		Small polyp forceps	1
	Criles	2			

SET • Neurology, Craniotomy

USE • Craniotomy, burr holes, acoustic neuromas, tumors, aneurysm, subdural hematoma, epidural hematoma

Instrument Index	Item(s)	PAR
Knife handles	#3	3
	#7	1
Suction tips	6 French Frazier	2
	8 French	2
	9 French	2
	10 French	2
	12 French	2
	Stylets	3
Scissors	Metzenbaum, small	1
	Metzenbaum, regular	1
	Mayo, small curved	1
	Mayo, large curved	1
	Nurse's	1
Forceps	Bayonet, regular	4
	Bayonet, fine	1
	Bayonet, cup	1
	9″ Potts	
	Adson, toothed	2
	Large ring	1
	Small ring	1
	Bipolar	2

Retractors	6 ½″ Weitlaner	2
	Sharp	
	Four-prong rakes, large	2
	Cushing	
	Weitlaner, curved	2
	Jansen	1
	Malleable brain	10
Elevators	Small periosteal	1
	Hoen	2
	Langenbeck	2
	Frazier, short	1
	Frazier, long	1
	Freer, wide	1
Bone instruments	Curette, small	1
	45 Kerrison 3 mm	1
	Large pituitary	1
	Leksell, small	1
	Leksell, medium	1
	Duckbill	1
	Rongeur, small	1
Clamps	Raney clip appliers	3
	Hemostats, straight	2
	Mosquitoes, straight	8
	Mosquitoes, curved	8
	Allises	16
	Kochers	2
	Kochers, large	2
	Towel clips, small	8
	Towel clips, large	8
Hemoclip appliers	Medium	2
	Small	2
	Sponge stick	1
Needle holders	7″ Dural, fine	2
	5″ Mayo-Hegar	2
	7″ Mayo-Hegar	2

Continued

Neurology, Craniotomy—cont'd

Instrument Index	Item(s)	PAR
Miscellaneous	Tissue hook	1
	Hudson brace	1
	Cerebellar extension	1
	Large ventricular cannulae with stylet	1
	Webster irrigation cannulae	1
	Gigli saw guide	1
	Solution basin	1

SET • Neurology, Laminectomy

USE • Laminectomy; disectomy; anterior and posterior cervical fusion; spinal fusion

Instrument Index	Item(s)	PAR
Knife handles	#3	3
	#7	1
Suction tips	12 Frazier	2
	8 Frazier	2
	Stylets	3
Scissors	8″ Mayo, straight	1
	Mayo, curved	1
	Metzenbaum, small	1
	Metzenbaum, regular	1
	Dandy ganglion	1
	Iris	1

Instrument Index	Item(s)	PAR
Forceps	Bayonet	2
	Bayonet, fine	1
	7″ Toothed	2
	Heavy toothed	2
	Adson, toothed	2
	Bipolar	2
Elevators	Periosteal, small	1
	Periosteal, large	1
	Langenbeck	2
	Cobbs, large	2
	#1 Penfield	1

Continued

Neurology, Laminectomy—cont'd

Instrument Index	Item(s)	PAR
	#2 Penfield	1
	#3 Penfield	1
	#4 Penfield	1
	Frazier, short	1
	Frazier, long	1
	Freer, wide	1
	Woodson	1
Bone instruments	Adson, rongeur	1
	Leksell, small	1
	Leksell, medium	1
	Leksell, large	1
	Straight pituitary, small	1
	Straight pituitary, large	1
	Up pituitary	1
	Down pituitary	1
	Hoen disc with teeth	1
Kerrisons	6″ 3 mm 45 degree angled	1
	6″ 5 mm 45 degree angled	1
	8″ 3 mm 45 degree angled	1
	8″ 5 mm 45 degree angled	1
	Right angled up	1
	Right angled down	1
	Horsley bone biter	1
	Ring curette	1

	Small reverse angle curette	1
	Curettes 0, 3, 5	3
Retractors	Weitlaner, short sharp	1
	Weitlaner, medium sharp	2
	Weitlaner, large sharp	2
	Army-Navy	2
	Four-prong rakes, large	2
	Scoville	1
	Blades	6
	Wing nuts	6
	Meyerding	1
	Beckman	1
	Nerve root	1
Clamps	Towel clips, small	8
	Towel clips, large	6
	Allises	10
	Kochers	2
	Hemostats, straight	2
	Mosquitoes, curved	6
	Mosquitoes, straight	6
	Ligament grasper	1
	Sponge stick	1
	Clip applier, medium	1
	Clip applier, small	1
Needle holders	7″ Dural, fine	2
	7″ Heavy	2

SET • Oral, Maxillofacial, Dental

USE • Teeth extraction, I & D mandible, arch bar placement, full mouth rehabilitation

Instrument Index	Item(s)	PAR
Extraction forceps	Universal 150	1
	Universal 151	1
	Cowhorn 89	1
	Cowhorn 90	1
	Lower incisor	2
Retractors	Mouth prop	1
	Army-Navy	1
	Dental rake	1
	Minnesota	1
	Skin hooks	2
	Tongue depressor	1

Instrument Index	Item(s)	PAR
Chisels	Small	1
	Single bibevel	1
	Gouge	1
Elevators	Short	1
	Straight	2
	Crane	1
	Miller	2
	Cameron	1
Bone instruments	Small single-action rongeur	1
	Mallet	2

	#4 Molt	1
	Seldon	1
	#9 Periosteal	1
	Freer	1
	Joseph	1
	Root tip pick	1
	Double-ended curette	1
	Bone file	1
Scissors	Nurse's	1
	Metzenbaum	1
	Doctor's	1
	Wire cutter	1
Needle holders	Wire twister	1
	Gold handle	1
	Plastic	1
Clamps	Hemostats, straight	2
	Mosquitoes	2
	Allises	2
	Kelly	1
	Kochers	2
	Crile	1
	Towel clips	3
Forceps	Dental	1
	Adson	1
	Tooth	1
	#3 Knife	1
Miscellaneous	Suction #10 Frazier	2
	Stylet	1
	Solution basin	1
	Tubex syringe	1

SET • Oral, Maxillofacial, Endoscopic

USE • Transmandibular joint (TMJ) replacement or revision

Instrument Index	Item(s)	PAR
Hook	1.5 mm	1
Scissors	6 ¼″ Mixter	1
Forceps	1.3 mm biopsy	1
	Alligator	1
Needle holder	Webster	1
Clamps	3 ½″ Nonpenetrating towel	4
	5 ½″ Nonpenetrating towel	2
	6″ Allis tissue with 4 × 5 teeth	2
	5 ½″ Hemostat, curved	2
	Mosquitoes, curved	2
	Mosquitoes, straight	1
Knife handle	#3, short	1
Miscellaneous	Obturator, dull	2
	Obturator, sharp	5
	2.5 mm trocar sheath	2
	3.2 mm trocar sheath	1
	2.5 mm cannula sheath	2

1.8 mm sheath	1		
Adaptors	2		
Rachet mouth prop	1		
Silastic tubing	1		
Solution basin	1		
Aluminum cup	2		

Video	30 degree scope, 1.9 mm	1
	30 degree scope, 2.4 mm	1
	Scope cover	1
	Camera	1

SET • Oral, Maxillofacial, Osteotomy

USE • Mandibular and maxilla fractures, geneoplasty, ORIF maxilla, TMJ

Instrument Index	Item(s)	PAR
Elevators	Right angled, downward	3
	Right angled, upward	1
Retractors	Army-Navy	2
	Senn	2
	Three-prong rake	2
	Ribbon	5
	Self-retaining coronoid Kelly with chain	1
	Tongue	2
	Mouth gag	1
	Rubber shods	2

Instrument Index	Item(s)	PAR
	Mouth prop with chain	1
	Mandibular body	1
Scissors	Nurse's	1
	Suture	1
	Metzenbaum, baby	1
	Wire cutters	1
Forceps	Smooth	1
	Dental	1
	Adson, toothed	2
	Adson-Brown	2
	DeBakey	1
	#3 Knife handle	2

Miscellaneous	#3 Knife handle, long	1
	Mosquitoes	5
	Hemostats, curved	4
	Kochers	2
	Allises	5
	Bone holding forceps	2
	Kellys	2
	Criles	2
	Towel clips, large	5
	Towel clips, small	2
	#10 Frazier	2
	Stylet	1
	Meniscus, single guarded	1
	Brown scissors	2
	Ravdin needle holder	2
	Crilewood	2
	Nasal Freer	1
	Angular periosteal elevator	1
	Woodson elevator	1
	Anterior border stripper	1
	Bone file	1
	Bone hook	1
	Rongeur	1
	Mallet	1
	Right-angled gouge	1
	Right and left row Kelly disimpaction forceps	2
	Double-ended curette	2
	Nerve hook	1
	Carpule syringe	1

Continued

Oral, Maxillofacial, Osteotomy—cont'd

Instrument Index	Item(s)	PAR
	Webster cannula	2
	Caliper	1
	Ruler	1
	Chuck key	1

Instrument Index	Item(s)	PAR
T-Bars	#8 Straight	1
	#6 Straight	1
	#4 Straight	1
	#6 Curved	1

SET • Orthopedics, Hand and Foot

USE • Carpal tunnel, ORIF radius, ankle fractures, toe amputations, ORIF wrist, replacement hand joint, tendon transfer, triple arthrodesis, wrist arthroscopy, ulnar nerve transfer, wrist fusion with bone graft

Instrument Index	Item(s)	PAR
Retractors	Baby rakes	2
	Skin hooks	2
	3″ Rakes, small	2
	Three-prong rakes, large	2
	Small right angle	2
	Army-Navy	2
	Weitlaner, small	1
	Weitlaner, medium	1
	Bunion	2
	Baby Hohmans	2
	Heis	2
	Senn	2
	Lami spreader, small	1
Forceps	Adson, toothed	2
	Adson-Brown	1
	Tooth	2
	Smooth	1

Continued

Orthopedics, Hand and Foot—cont'd

Instrument Index	Item(s)	PAR
	Adson, smooth	1
	7″ DeBakey	2
Scissors	Doctor's	1
	Iris	1
	Nurse's	1
	Bandage	1
	Brown	1
	Metzenbaum, baby	1
	Metzenbaum, regular	1
	Pin/Wire cutter	1
	Tenotomy	1
Miscellaneous	#10 Frazier suction, short	2
	Ruler	1

Instrument Index	Item(s)	PAR
	Nerver hooks	1
Scalpel handles	#3 Knife	7
	#7 Knife	1
Clamps	Jacksons	2
	Mosquitoes, curved	6
	Mosquitoes, straight	6
	Hemostats, curved	6
	Hemostats, straight	6
	Allises	4
	Kochers	4
	Kellys	2
	Sponge sticks	3
	Towel clips, small	4
	Towel clips, regular	2

	Jakes	2
Needle holders	Mayo, regular	1
	Small plastic	2
Elevators	Small key	1
	Freer	1
	Cobb, small	1
	Curettes, variety	6
	Bone cutter, small	1
	Needlenose pliers	1
	Metal mallet, small	1
	Drill bit box set	1
	Rongeur, small double action	1
	Rongeur, baby single-action curved	1
	Ear curette	1
Hand osteotomes	Three-eighths ($\frac{3}{8}$)	1
	Three-sixteenths ($\frac{3}{16}$)	1
	Five-sixteenths ($\frac{5}{16}$)	1
	One-fourth ($\frac{1}{4}$)	1
	One-eighth ($\frac{1}{8}$)	1

SET • Orthopedics, Total Hip

USE • I & D of one hip, total hip, revision hip, ORIF hip, I & D thigh, pelvis fracture, IM rod, acetabular fracture

Instrument Index	Item(s)	PAR
Retractors	Weitlaner	2
	Beckman	2
	Deaver, broad	2
	Deaver, narrow	2
	Cobra, curved	1
	Cobra, straight	1
	Israeli rake	2
	Bennett	2
	Hibb, large	2
	Hibb, small	2
	Army-Navy	2

Instrument Index	Item(s)	PAR
Suction	#11 Frazier, long	1
Forceps	Ferris	2
	Long smooth	1
	Long tooth	1
	Short tooth	2
	Adson, toothed	2
Scissors	Nurse's	1
	Suture	1
	Mayo	1
	Bandage	1
	Metzenbaum	1

	Metzenbaum, long	1
	Needle holder	4
Scalpel handles	#3	2
	#3, long	3
Clamps	Hemostat, curved	10
	Hemostat, straight	5
	Kellys	10
	Kellys, long	2
	Kochers	6
	Allises	6
	Criles	2
Bone instruments	Mallet	1
	Bone cutter	1
	Rongeur, large	1
	Rongeur, small	1
	Bone hook	1
	Cobb, large	1
	Wire cutter	1
	Plier	1
	Bone tamp	1
	Sweetheart clamp	1
	Key or Scott McCracken	1
	Towel clip, large	10
	Drill bit box	1
	Sponge stick	4
	Ruler	1
Osteotome	¼ Straight	1
	¾ Straight	1
	½ Curved	1

SET • Orthopedics, Total Knee

USE • Total knee, I & D knee, revision knee, patellar fracture, tibial fracture, ORIF tibia, high tibial osteotomy

Instrument Index	Item(s)	PAR
Retractors	Four-prong rake, dull	2
	Four-prong rake, sharp	2
	Weitlaner, medium	2
	Army-Navy	2
	Hohmann, sharp	1
	Hohmann, dull	1
	"Z"	2
Forceps	Ferris Smith	2
	Adson, toothed	2
	Adson-Brown	1
	Tooth	2

Instrument Index	Item(s)	PAR
Scissors	Bandage	1
	Mayo	1
	Suture	1
	Metzenbaum	1
	Nurse's	1
Clamps	Hemostat, curved	5
	Hemostat, straight	5
	Kochers	8
	Kellys	6
	Allises	8
	Towel clips	10

Scalpel handles	#3	3
	#7	1
Suctions	Stylet	1
	#10 Frazier	2
	Sponge stick	4
Bone instruments	Key or Scott McCracken, large	1
	Cobb, medium	1
	½ Key elevator	1
	Bone tamp	1
	Bone hook	1
	Curettes	4
	Pliers	1
	Rongeur, small (double action)	1
	Rongeur, large	1
	Bone clamp, sweetheart	1
	Box drill bits	1
	Teflon mallet	1
	Lami spreader, large	1
Osteotomes	Straight ¼	1
	Straight ⅝	1
	Curved ¼	1
	Straight ¾	1
Miscellaneous	Needle holder	4
	Ruler	1

SET • Otorhinolaryngology, Radical

USE • Neck dissection, parotid dissection, thyroid dissection, larynx dissection, pharynx dissection, composite neck dissection

Instrument Index	Item(s)	PAR
Retractors	Weitlaner	1
	Army-Navy	2
	Senn	2
	Vein	2
	Short skin hooks	2
	Double prong skin hooks	2
	Double skin hooks, wide width	4
	Four-prong rakes	2
	Six-prong rakes	2

Instrument Index	Item(s)	PAR
	Side biting mouth gag	1
	Kelly Richardson, small	1
	Kelly Richardson, large	1
	Green	2
	Deaver, small narrow	2
	#6 Deaver	1
	#7 Deaver	1
	Cheek	2
	Lagenbeck	2
	Malleable, small	1
	Malleable, medium	1

	Malleable, large	1
	#3	1
	#7	1
Forceps	Adson, toothed	1
	Bayonet	1
	6″ DeBakey	2
	Adson-Brown	2
	Bishoo Harmon, wide teeth	2
	Walter, gold handle	1
	Lorenz with teeth	2
	Adson, bipolar	1
	Brown	2
Elevators	Freer	1
	Cottle	1
	Joseph	1
	Periosteal, medium	1
	Obegezzer, curved	1
	Nerve hook	1
Clamps	Hemostats, curved	10
	Hemostats, straight	6
	Mosquitoes, curved	20
	Allises	10
	Kellys	4
	Kochers	4
	Criles, fine	4
	7″ Gemini clamps, fine tip	2
	8″ Gemini clamps, fine tip	2
	Gemini clamps, fine tip	2
	Laheys	6
	Babcocks	6

Continued

Otorhinolaryngology, Radical—cont'd

Instrument Index	Item(s)	PAR
	Jackson	1
	McCabe dissectors	2
	Jakes	2
	Towel clips, small	16
	Dandies	3
	Adson, curved hemostat	2
Scissors	Metzenbaum, baby	2
	Metzenbaum	1
	Mayo, large	1
	Nurse's	2
	Iris	1
	Tenotomy	1
	Tenotomy, long	1
	Mayo, small	1
	Rhytidectomy	1
	Mallis	1
	Webster	2
	7″ Serot	4
Suctions	6 mm Frazier	2
	8 mm Frazier	2
	10 mm Frazier	2

12 mm Frazier	2	Miscellaneous	Sponge stick	1
Mastoid	1		Tongue depressor	1
Andrew Pononon pediatric Yankauer	2		Tracheal hook	1
			Tracheal spreader	1

SET • Otorhinolaryngology, Tonsil

USE • Tonsillectomy

Instrument Index	Item(s)	PAR
Mouth gags	Crow-Davis	1
	Blades, small, medium, large	3
	Melvor	1
Knives	#7 Handle	1
	Fisher	1
	Douglas flag	1
Clamps	Kellys	3
	Criles	3
	Allises, short	2
	Allises, long curved	2

Instrument Index	Item(s)	PAR
	Towel clips, small	4
	Sponge stick	1
Scissors	Metzenbaum, regular	1
	Doctor's scissors, long	1
Forceps	Bayonet	1
	Small cup	1
	Tenaculum	1
Suction	Yankauer	1
Curettes	Adenoid, reverse curved	1

Miscellaneous instruments	Tongue depressor	1
	Uvula retractor	1
	Tonsil snare	1
	Pillar dissector	1
	Monopolar, curved	1
	Cups	2
	Medicine glass	1
	Solution basin	1
Needle holders	Medium	2

SET • Otorhinolaryngology, Tracheostomy

USE • Tracheostomy

Instrument Index	Item(s)	PAR
Retractors	Weitlaner	1
	Army-Navy	2
	Senn	2
	Vein	2
	Skin hooks, long	2
	Skin hooks, short	2
	Green	2
Forceps	DeBakey	2
	Adson, toothed	2
	Bayonet	1
	Lorenz gold	2
Suctions	Tonsil	1
	Mastoid	1
	Frazier	2
Scalpel handles	#3	2
	#7	1
Scissors	Metzenbaum, baby	2
	Mayo	2
	Nurse's	1
	Iris	1
	Tenotomy	1

Clamps	Mosquito hemostats, curved	10
	Hemostats, curved	10
	Allises	5
	Kellys	5
	Jacksons	2
	Towel clips	6
	Dandies	3
Needle holders	7″ Mayo-Hegar	2
	Brown, plastic	2
Miscellaneous	Tongue depressor	1
	Tracheal hook	1
	Tracheal spreader	1
	Cups	2
	Solution basin	1

SET • Thoracic, Mediastinoscopy

USE • Mediastinoscopy

Instrument Index	Item(s)	PAR
Retractors	Cushing vein	2
	Army-Navy	2
	Senn	2
	Skin hooks	2
	Weitlaner	1
	Lehey	2
Miscellaneous	Mediastinoscope	2
	Light cable	1
	Bovie cord	1
	Biopsy forceps	2
	Aspiration needles	2
	Insulated bovie suction	1
	Yankauer	1
Scalpel handles	#3, short	1
Scissors	Metzenbaum, regular	1
	Suture	1
Needle holders	7″ Vascular	2
	7″ Mayo-Hegar	2
Forceps	DeBakey, medium	2
	10″ Long smooth	1

	5″ Short smooth	1
	Russians, long	1
	5″ Tooth	1
	Adson	2
Clamps	Mosquitoes, curved	4
	Hemostats, curved	4
	Hemostats, straight	2
	Criles	4
	Allises	4
	Allises, long	2
	Kellys, long	2
	Mixtures	2
	Sponge stick	1
	Towel clips, small	4
	Towel clips, large	6

SET • Thoracic, Thoracotomy, Major

USE • Chest wall resection, pulmonary resection, lobectomy, segmentectomy, Wedge resection, pneumonectomy, bilateral bullectomies, volume reduction, pectus excavatum repair

Instrument Index	Item(s)	PAR
Retractors	Child chest	1
	Finochetto Burford	1
	Blades	4
	Whisks	1
	Malleable, medium	1
	Kelly Richardson, large	1
	Kelly Richardson, medium	1
	Kelly Richardson, small	1
	Kelly Richardson, baby	1
	Cushing vein	2
	Army-Navy	2
	Weitlaner, dull	1
	Three-prong rakes, sharp	2
Clip appliers	Long, large	2
	Long, medium	2
Suctions	Pool	1
	Yankauer	2
	Pediatric Yankauer	1
Knife handles	#3, short	2
	#3, long	2
	#7	1
	Beaver 2000	1

	Gigli saw	1
	Gigli saw handle	2
	Nerve hook	1
	Rumel	1
Needle holders	7″ Sarot	2
	8″ Vascular	2
	9″ Vascular	2
	Mayo-Hegar	4
	Sternal	2
	French eye, long	2
Scissors	Potts	1
	Metzenbaum	1
	Metzenbaum, long	2
	Metzenbaum, extra long	1
	Short heavy straight	1
	Wire cutter/sternal	1
	Long suture	1
Forceps	8 ¼″ Diamond tip	2
	7″ DeBakey	2
	10″ DeBakey	2
	12″ DeBakey	2
	Russian	2
	Adson	2
	8″ Toothed	2
Clamps	Mosquitoes, curved	4
	Mosquitoes, straight	4
	Hemostats, curved	6
	Hemostats, straight	6
	Kellys	2
	Kellys, long	2
	Kochers	6
	Kochers, long	2
	Allises	4
	Allis, long	2
	Allis, Judd	4

Continued

Thoracic, Thoracotomy, Major—cont'd

Instrument Index	Item(s)	PAR
	Criles	4
	Crile, extra long	2
	Mixtures	2
	Mixtures, fine tip	2
	Mixtures, snub nose	2
	Babcock, long	2
	Bronchus	2
	DeBakey, angled	2
	DeBakey clamp	2
	DeBakey, straight	2
	Harkin	1
	Lorenz, angled	1

Instrument Index	Item(s)	PAR
	Tubing	3
	Satinsky, large	1
	Satinsky, medium	1
	Satinsky, small	1
	Fogarty, small angled	1
	Fogarty, small straight	1
	Duvall	2
	Lovelace	1
	Spoon	1
	Sponge stick	4
	Towel clips	8

SET • Urology, Urology Tray, Robotic

USE • Robotic radical prostatectomy, sacrocolpopexy with sling and pyeloplasty

Instrument Index	Item(s)	PAR
Tray	Robotic instrument	1
Forceps	Bipolar Maryland	1
	Cadiere	1

Instrument Index	Item(s)	PAR
Needle driver	Large	1
	Suture cut	1
Scissors	Monopolar, curved	1
	Round tip	1

SET • Vascular, Hickman

USE • Port access, Hickman placement, portacath placement, phoresis catheter placement, catheter removals

Instrument Index	Item(s)	PAR
Retractors	Weitlaner, blunt	2
	Mastoid, small	1
	Three-prong rake, blunt	2
	Three-prong rake, sharp	2
	Maison	2
	Vein	2
	Army-Navy	2
	Band	2
Scissors	Metzenbaum, regular	1
	Metzenbaum, baby	1
	Church	1
	Nurse's	1
	Suture	1
Forceps	Short smooth	2
	Short tooth	2
	Adson, toothed	2
	Vascular, short	2
	7″ Vascular	2
Clamps	Mosquitoes, curved	10
	Mosquitoes, straight	4

	Hemostat, curved	6
	Hemostat, straight	6
	Jacksons	2
	Kellys	2
	Kelly, long	1
	Allises	2
	Beck	1
	Towel clips, small	6
	Crile, long	1
	Sponge stick	1
Suction tips	Plastic	1
	Frazier	1
Scalpel handles	#3	2
	#7	1
Miscellaneous	Probe	1
	Groove director	1
	Webster cannula	1
	Coronary dilators (1.0, 1.5, 2.0, 2.5, 3.0)	5
	Solution basin	1
	Cups	3
	Needle holder	2
	Webster	2
	7″ Mayo-Hegar	2

SET • Vascular, Major

USE • Abdominal aneurysm, kidney transplant, kidney-pancreas transplant

Instrument Index	Item(s)	PAR
Retractors Deavers	Shallow	2
	Deep	2
	Broad	3
	Cushing vein	2
	Army-Navy	2
	Kelly Richardson, large	1
	Weitlaner	3
	Beckman, deep sharp	1
	Malleable	1
	Bands	2

Instrument Index	Item(s)	PAR
Suctions	#9 and #10 Frazier, short	2
	#11 Frazier, long	2
	Nerve hook	1
	Groove director	1
	Probe	1
	Ruler	1
Hemoclip appliers	Small	1
	Medium	2
	Large	2

Scalpel handles	#3	3
	#7	1
	#3, long	1
Scissors	Metzenbaum, regular	1
	Metzenbaums, long	2
	Metzenbaum, extra long	1
	Long suture	1
	Nurse's	1
	Suture	1
	Church	1
	7″ Potts	1
	Lincoln	1
Forceps	7″ Vascular	2
	9″ Atragrip	3
	Long smooth	2
	Adson, toothed	2
	Russians	2
	7″ Titanium rhoton	2
	Short toothed	2
	Blue burners, long	2
Clamps	Jacksons	2
	Mosquitoes, curved	4
	Mosquitoes, straight	8
	Hemostats, curved	6
	Hemostats, straight	6
	Kellys	2
	Kellys, long	2
	Kochers	6
	Allises	6
	Allises, long	2
	Criles	6
	Mixtures	6
	Sponge sticks	2
	Towel clips	12
	Crafoord, Shod	2

Continued

Vascular, Major—cont'd

Instrument Index	Item(s)	PAR
	Crafoord, super	1
	Fogarty, long straight	2
	Fogarty, long angled	2
	Aortic	4
	Satinsky, super flatback	1
	Satinsky, super curved back	1
	Beck	2
	Cooley	1
	Fogarty, short straight	4
	Fogarty, short curved	4
	Bent handle aortic	3
Needle holders	10″ Vascular, long	4
	9″ Mayo-Hegar	4
	6″ Mayo-Hegar	1
	French eye, long	2
	French eye	2
	Serot	2
Vascular instruments	Potts scissors, small	2
	Iris scissors, small	2
	5″ Vascular, fine forceps	4
	Castroviejo needle holders	2

Vascular bulldog clamps	5
Cannulae	2
Coronary bulldogs	3
Mueller bulldog, straight	2
Mueller bulldog, curved	1
Coronary dilators	5

SET • Vascular, Minor

USE • Above the knee, below the knee, AV fistula graft, carotid endarterectomy

Instrument Index	Item(s)	PAR
Retractors	Deaver, shallow	2
	Army-Navy	2
	Bands	3
	Cushing vein	2
	Kelly Richardson	1
	Thyroid rakes	2
	Weitlaner, dull	2
	Weitlaner, small dull	1
	Henley	1
	Henley blades	2
	Beckman, dull deep	1
	Oschner	1
Suctions	#12 Frazier, short	1
	#4 Frazier, short	1
Hemoclip appliers	Small	2
	Medium	2
Miscellaneous	Nerve hook	1
	Freer elevator	1
	Ruler	1
	#3 Knife handles	2
	#7 Knife handle	1
Scissors	Metzenbaum, regular	1
	Metzenbaum, long	1
	Church	1

	7″ Potts	1
	Nurse's	1
	Suture	1
	Suture, large	1
Forceps	Short smooth	2
	Adson, toothed	2
	7″ Atragrips	2
	7″ Titanium	2
	Rat tooth	2
Clamps	Jacksons	4
	Mosquitoes, curved	4
	Mosquitoes, straight	8
	Hemostats, curved	6
	Hemostats, straight	4
	Kellys, short	4
	Kochers	4
	Allises	6
	Towel clips	12
	Criles	2
	Mixtures	2
	Sponge stick	1
	Beck	1
	Cooley	2
	Kellys, long	1
	Fogarty, curved	4
	Fogarty, straight	4
	Crafoord, super	1
	Rumel	1
Carotids	Large	1
	Small	1
	Special carotid clamps	2
Fine vascular instruments	Potts scissors, small	2
	Iris scissors, small	2
	5″ Vascular, fine forceps	4

Continued

Vascular, Minor—cont'd

Instrument Index	Item(s)	PAR
	Castroviejo needle holder	2
	Coronary bulldogs	2
	Cannulae	2
	Vascular clamps, small	5
	Coronary dilators	5
	Mueller bulldog, straight	1
	Mueller bulldog, curved	1
Needle holders	9″ Mayo-Hegar	2
	6″ Mayo-Hegar	2
	Serot	2
	Ravdin	2

Glossary

Angled: Bent, not straight (e.g., in Potts scissors)

Atraumatic: Not having a crushing or biting effect on tissue

Bayonet: A blade that is offset from the axis of the handle

Chisel: A wedge-like instrument with a blade for cutting or chipping

Clamp: Device used to hold an object in a fixed position; occluder for blood vessels and other organs

Clip: A metal fastener for joining or approximating the edges of a wound

Curet (curette): A spoon-shaped instrument for scraping or cutting

Curved: Bent, or continuously deviating from a straight line, as in a curved blade or handle

Dilator: An instrument used for stretching or enlarging an opening or tube

Dissector: An instrument used in dissection

Dull: Blunt; not sharp

Elevator: An instrument used for lifting or retaining

Fine: Having thin or slender jaws or tips; fine scissors, forceps, or clamps have very narrow tips; used for delicate or small, precise procedures (e.g., vascular surgery, plastic surgery, infertility procedures, neurosurgery)

Forceps: A two-bladed instrument for handling tissues and dressings

Heavy: Having broad jaws or tips (e.g., scissors, forceps) that can be used for thick or tough tissue

Internal staplers: Specialized staples used in place of sutures in open surgical procedures

Knife: A blade with a sharp edge used for cutting

Mallet: A hammer-like instrument used for striking objects

Minimally invasive endoscopic instruments: Instruments used through small incisions to remove, cut, suture, grasp, or inflate (e.g., for laparoscopic and robotic surgeries)

Micro: Small, narrow, or delicate

Needle holder: An instrument used to grasp the suturing device

Osteotome: A chisel-like instrument used for cutting or marking bone

Retractor: An instrument used for grasping, retaining, or holding back tissue for surgical exposure

Rongeur: A biting instrument used for cutting tough tissue or bone

Saw: A notched blade used for cutting

Scissors: A cutting instrument with two shearing blades

Self-retaining: Capable of being placed into a fixed position (e.g., a self-retaining clamp)

Serrations: The small grooves seen on the edges or tips of an instrument; can be vertical or horizontal

Sharp: Implies a point tip when referring to a retractor, such as a rake

Smooth: Without teeth; may be serrated, but does not have a projection to penetrate tissue

Snare: An instrument with a wire loop for removing a tissue growth by encircling it and closing the loop

Suction tip: A hollow tube-like instrument that is attached to a vacuum for suction

Surgical instrument: A specifically designed tool or device for performing specific actions of surgery or operations (e.g., modifying biological tissue or providing access for viewing it)

Surgical power tools: Instruments used mostly for small and large bone procedures; functions include drilling, shaving, reaming, cutting, tunneling, and fixation

Suture: A string-like device, usually made of catgut or nylon, used for joining or approximating tissue (e.g., in wound closure)

Toothed: Having small notches or projections used to grasp tissue and prevent the instrument from slipping

Traumatic: Having a crushing or biting effect on tissue

References

Fuller JK: *Surgical technology: principles and practice*, ed 5, Philadelphia, 2010, Saunders.

Hutchisson BA, Phippen ML, Wells MA: *Review of perioperative nursing*, Philadelphia, 2000, Saunders.

Illustrated medical dictionary, ed 31, Philadelphia, 2007, Saunders.

Miller-Keane, O'Toole MT (ed): *Miller-Keane encyclopedia and dictionary of medicine, nursing, and allied health* (revised reprint), ed 7, Philadelphia, 2005, Saunders.

Phippen M, Ulmer B, Wells M: *Competency for safe patient care during operative and invasive procedures*, Denver, 2009, Competency & Credentialing Institute (CCI).

Phippen ML, Wells MA: *Patient care during operative and invasive procedures*, Philadelphia, 2000, Saunders.

Phippen ML, Wells MA: *Perioperative nursing practice*, Philadelphia, 1994, Saunders.

Smith MF, Stehn JL: *Basic surgical instrumentation*, Philadelphia, 1993, Saunders.

Tighe SM: *Instrumentation for the operating room: a photographic manual*, ed 7, St. Louis, 2007, Mosby.

Index

C

D

E

F

G

H

M

N

O

T

U

V

W

Y